"Drs. Sandy and Todd Severin have done much more than write a book: In *TriEnergetics* they've created a sensible anlp you turn your life toward vibrant health a d-able information, and a carefully mapp th mind, body, and nutrition, *TriEnergetics* co th changes can only come about through a gentle yet thorough reorientation of the way we live.

—Norman Fischer, former Abbot of the San Francisco Zen Center, founder of and teacher at the Everyday Zen Foundation, and author of *Taking Our Places: The Buddhist Path to Truly Growing Up*

"Health is more than absence of disease. Drs. Todd and Sanford Severin are to be congratulated for broadening the concept of health to optimal physical and mental well-being. The principles and techniques described in *TriEnergetics*, represent an excellent holistic approach to achieving optimal health through meditation for the mind, physical exercise for the body and good nutrition."

—Scott S. Lee, MD

"*TriEnergetics* is an uplifting program that goes beyond the 'how-to' and into the "why" that is the foundation of self-improvement. Finally, there is a refreshing approach that recognizes the importance of the mind and spirit in the health of the body."

—Steve Bylsma, MD

"The effect of stress on our health and disease is underemphasized in western medicine. *TriEnergetics* is a program that will help you regain control of that vital process. *TriEnergetics* is essential for obtaining a healthy outlook on life."

—Neil Okamura, DO

"*TriEnergetics* should be an inspiration to us all. True health can only be achieved if we appreciate and nurture the link between the mind and body. This program shows us how to do just that."

—Valerie Schneider, MD

"*TriEnergetics* emphasizes health of the mind and spirit as well as the body, while teaching healthy dietary as well as exercise habits. Only this kind of integrated approach can achieve true, lasting vitality."

—Daniel A. Brinton, MD

"The multifactorial nature of disease and aging dictates a multifactorial approach to health and longevity. This is the cornerstone principle of *TriEnergetics*, well articulated and outlined here by the Drs. Severin, who live what they teach."

—Shirin Barez, MD

"This is the owners guide for your body! *TriEnergetics* provides a wealth of information on physical and emotional health, and establishes a framework for incorporating sound dietary, nutritional, exercise and stress reduction practices into a daily program for well-being."

—Kevin Beadles, MD

"Drs. Severin bring together a range of personal and scholarly expertise and practice in modern medicine, nutrition, exercise, and Eastern philosophy to this balanced and satisfying approach to health and well-being."

—Ray Gariano, MD

"As a primary care physician, I see patient after patient with problems that Western lifestyles create, including heart disease, diabetes, palpitations, abdominal pains, panic attacks and many others. The approach that Drs. Todd and Sanford Severin advocate in *TriEnergetics* is what I have found most helpful in caring for patients with these problems."

—Jim Eichel, MD

TriEnergetics

Balancing
Nutrition, Exercise
& Mindfulness
for Lasting Wellness

SANFORD L. SEVERIN, MD
TODD D. SEVERIN, MD

New Harbinger Publications, Inc.

Publisher's Note

Distributed in Canada by Raincoast Books.

Copyright © 2005 by Sanford Severin and Todd Severin
New Harbinger Publications, Inc.
5674 Shattuck Avenue
Oakland, CA 94609
www.newharbinger.com

Previously published in 2002 by Opitma Press.

Cover design by Amy Shoup; Text design by Michele Waters-Kermes;
Acquired by Jess O'Brien; Edited by Jessica Beebe

Printed in the United States of America. All Rights Reserved.

Library of Congress Cataloging-in-Publication Data

Severin, Sanford L., 1934-
  Trienergetics : balancing nutrition, exercise, and mindfulness for lasting wellness /
Sandford L. Severin, and Todd D. Severin.
      p. cm.
  Includes bibliographical references.
  ISBN 1-57224-445-3
  1. Health. 2. Physical fitness. 3. Nutrition. 4. Exercise. I. Severin, Todd D., 1963- II.
Title.
  RA776.S4838 2005
  613.7—dc22
                                2005027989
07 06 05

10 9 8 7 6 5 4 3 2 1

First printing

We want to dedicate this book to our loving wives, without whose love and support this project would never have seen the light of day.

For Joy and Corinne

Contents

PART 2
The TriEnergetics Program

Acknowledgments

This book would not have been possible without the significant contributions of a number of people. We are indebted to each and every one of them for their assistance and guidance.

In particular, we'd like to thank Joy Severin for all her hard work in making this dream come to reality; Corinne for her loving support and encouragement; Don Gerrard for his editorial advice, guidance, and critique; Susan Sparrow of Tenacity Press for production assistance and guidance; Claudia Moose, ATC, for exercise training; Pam Wilson, RD, for nutritional guidance; Ted Zeff, Ph.D., for stress reduction techniques; Don Flory, Ph.D., for deep breathing techniques; Norm Fisher, abbot of the San Francisco Zen Center, for peace of mind and meditation counseling; and John Estes for his wonderful illustrations.

preface

A New Health Paradigm

Take a long, hard look at your life.

If you don't look as good as you would like to look, feel as good as you would like to feel, or have the energy and enthusiasm for life that you really want to have, this book is for you. If you have tried to diet and regained the weight, started an exercise program and failed, been unsuccessful in curbing your stress, or attempted to take control over your life only to watch that control slip away, this book is for you. In fact, this book offers everyone the opportunity to jump-start their lives with better health, energy, and vitality by following our revolutionary lifestyle plan—the TriEnergetics program.

TriEnergetics is different than any other health, diet, or exercise book you will find on the market today. TriEnergetics represents a whole new concept of wellness; it's a six-week program that will change your life.

ENERGY IS LIFE

We've designed the TriEnergetics program with one express goal: to help you balance the three key energies of your life—the natural energies of your body, your mind, and your nourishment.

 Body energy refers to all of the energies necessary to keep your body alive. This includes the energy needed for skeletal muscle movement, circulation, hormonal regulation, immune balance, breathing, and digestion.

 Mind energy refers to the process of thought. It involves not only the energy required to create the thought but also how the thought itself can affect your body.

 Nourishment energy refers to the health and vitality derived from the foods you eat. Ultimately, this energy is responsible for sustaining mind energy and body energy.

Each of these three vital energies is essential for maximum wellness. You can't exercise your way to good health while ignoring your nourishment needs or your level of stress, and likewise, you can't meditate or eat your way to good health while ignoring your body's need for movement and exercise. Only by balancing the three key energies of the body can you achieve total wellness. The TriEnergetics program will help you do just that.

THE IMPORTANCE OF WHOLENESS

Your body is a little universe, consisting of more than ten billion cells organized into tissues, organs, and systems, all having the innate ability to regulate themselves and maintain internal order. For your body to function at its peak level of health and harmony, every organ system, muscle, nerve, sense organ, and gland—even every cell—must be in balance.

To accomplish this delicate balance, the body uses finely tuned feedback loops that interconnect every aspect of your being. On every level—from the workings of a single cell to the functioning of your organ systems—your physiology is regulated by an internal flow of hormones, electrical signals, growth factors, and neurotransmitters, connecting each part of your body to every other part. Anything that disrupts one system will disrupt the others too.

Thousands of years ago, Taoist sages understood the fundamental wholeness of the body. Much of their early writings concentrated on the importance of balancing and harmonizing the energies of the mind and the body. They knew the mind and the body were interconnected, and they recognized that what affects one will undoubtedly affect the other.

The holistic outlook of Taoist healers contrasts sharply with classical Western medicine, in which doctors compartmentalize the mind and the body and then subdivide the compartments. The ultimate result is the complete separation of the mind and body. If someone has emotional problems, he goes to a psychiatrist for therapy. If someone is obese, she goes on a diet to lose weight. If someone is flabby and has no muscle tone, he gets a personal trainer or a stair-climber and begins to exercise. Few Western doctors look at how the emotional problem is affecting the eating, or how the lack of exercise is contributing to the emotional problem, or how the person's nutritional state affects the whole body.

Like the Taoist sages, we believe in the wholeness of the body. If you don't eat well, your body will suffer and your thinking will be affected. If you don't get enough exercise, your body will deteriorate and stress will build up, affecting your mind. If you don't deal with your stress positively, your immune system will malfunction and your health will suffer. The body is one whole. Everything is connected.

TRIENERGETICS WILL BRING YOU BACK INTO BALANCE

Through our wellness seminars, classes, and workshops, we have learned that the key to developing a healthy body and mind is to respect the wholeness of your being. To do this, you must work with all three of your essential energies simultaneously and bring your body back into balance. This is the guiding principle of the TriEnergetics program.

This isn't an exercise book, a diet book, a weight loss book, or a stress reduction book. What makes TriEnergetics so different is that we don't just offer advice on what to eat or tips for a few exercises. TriEnergetics is a complete, balanced lifestyle plan designed to help you harmonize the three key energies of your body and, in the process, look better and feel years younger.

With the TriEnergetics program, you will no longer need to guess at what's necessary to live a healthy, energizing lifestyle. We have created an easy-to-follow six-week program that tells you exactly what you need to do each day of each week. Following this plan, you'll be amazed at how easy it is to make quantum changes in the way you look and feel.

Best of all, to get started, you don't need to make radical changes in your life. Each week, for six weeks, you only have to make a small change in your nourishment, your exercise, and your relaxation skills. Each weekly change builds upon the change you made the week before. That's why the program works. There is no pain and no sudden lifestyle changes. No major hurdles that you have to conquer. All you have to do is make a few small changes each week, and by the end of the six weeks, you'll be stunned at how far you've come and how easy it's been to get there. It's that simple.

Now there are no barriers standing between you and the healthy, energetic life you've been wanting to live. With the TriEnergetics program, you can move forward on the path of total wellness, improving your health, losing weight, and integrating your body and your mind.

Best of all, we will be your constant companions on your path toward looking better and feeling younger. Let us know how you're doing through our Web site at www.trienergetics.com. We will be there for you.

So let's get started. Have fun!

chapter 1

Look Better, Feel Younger Now!
It's Never Too Late to Start

We'd like to introduce you to one of the many people who have transformed their lives through TriEnergetics.

● Maria's Metamorphosis

Maria's life had fallen apart. Forty-four years old and a successful businesswoman, she'd spent years living a highly charged life. Married, an entrepreneur and a mother, she had been flourishing, maintaining her family, her career, and her personal life. The kids were healthy, the business was succeeding, and her relationship was stable. In her mind, things couldn't get any better. Maria felt that she was living the American dream.

Then her problems began. First came the nagging symptoms: the weakness in her left arm, the troubling distortions in her vision, and the persistent headaches. Months of medical examinations finally led her to face her ultimate fear: she was diagnosed with multiple sclerosis, a chronic and debilitating neurologic condition. Within months of her diagnosis, her husband of twenty-two years left her, saying that he didn't want to spend his life with an invalid. With her health and her personal life crashing down around her, Maria's business crumbled and teetered on the brink of bankruptcy. She was ill, frightened, angry, and very alone.

That was Maria's condition when she first came to our TriEnergetics program, sponsored by the hospital in her hometown. Maria silently slid into the back of the meeting room and sat down. Angry at her failing health and the collapse of her dream life, she folded her arms tightly across her chest and looked at us with a disbelieving glare that seemed to say, "Go on, make me well."

To make a long story short, we never did make Maria well. She did it herself.

At the beginning of the sixth week in the program, Maria approached us with tears in her eyes and an open heart. She was overwhelmed by the realization of how much her health had improved. Her multiple sclerosis symptoms had improved dramatically. She had altered her diet and incorporated the exercises and stress management techniques into her life. She now radiated energy. She felt so good that she enrolled in college, where her younger classmates could barely keep up with her.

Maria went from a state of disease—mentally, physically, and emotionally—to such a level of physical, nutritional, and emotional fitness that she developed what we call *dynamic energy*.

DYNAMIC ENERGY

Dynamic energy. These are two very powerful words, but what do they mean? Think for a moment. What would it mean to have dynamic energy? What would it be like to have a boundless enthusiasm for life, to flow through your life without tiring, to get all the things done that you have been putting off, to enjoy life to the fullest with your cup overflowing? Is this just a pipe dream?

We don't think so. We believe that it is your biological heritage to have dynamic energy. You were born with it. You are entitled to it. Dynamic energy is what naturally results from a healthy, integrated lifestyle that balances the three key energies of the body, the mind, and nourishment.

The problem is that the chaos of daily life takes its toll on you. Work gets in the way of exercising, family issues take over, stress builds to intolerable levels, you tend to move your body less and less while eating more. Your body begins to feel ill. Your mind runs in circles. The result of all this physical and mental strain is the loss of your natural energy.

As your energy fades, your lifestyle takes you farther and farther from wellness. You lose the delicate balance of the three energies and fall farther out of synchrony. Your emotions suffer, your psychological well-being suffers, and finally, your health suffers.

FINDING THE PATH

We've worked with countless people in our TriEnergetics seminars and workshops and have learned that it's possible to improve your health, your appearance, and your feeling of well-being so much that you will develop dynamic energy. You can regain control of your life and create a lifestyle that fosters health, balance, and the natural abundance of energy that lives inside of you.

Are you interested? Do you want to know what you have to do to get on the path to better health? Read on. We will show you the way. We will show you how you can look better, feel younger, and have fun doing it. In fact, you can feel better than you have ever felt in your life.

● Gerry: The Personification of Dynamic Energy

In some ways, Gerry is an ordinary guy. He's married, has children, owns a home, and walks his dog every day. But in other ways, Gerry is different. For starters, he runs five or six marathons a year. He skis avidly, runs six miles every day rain or shine, pumps iron three times a week, takes yearly canoe trips into the Canadian wilderness, loves to go for long hikes in the mountains, and works as a consulting engineer.

Maybe you aren't impressed. Not such a big deal. He's just a very active guy, right? Well, let's add one more bit of information. Gerry is eighty-three years old. Now what do you think?

And what would you think if we told you that thirteen years ago, Gerry was a stressed-out, overweight engineer who had suffered a heart attack at the age of seventy? Now are you impressed?

Here is a guy who has transformed his life. By incorporating the revolutionary principles of the TriEnergetics program, Gerry has become as addicted to good health as other people are to nicotine or chocolate. His latest goal, by the way, is to run a marathon on his hundredth birthday.

YOU CAN CREATE YOUR OWN DYNAMIC ENERGY

Is it really possible to make quantum changes, as Gerry did, in the way you look and feel? The answer is an enthusiastic yes!

We're not asking you to go out and run a marathon. You don't need this level of physical activity to generate wellness and dynamic energy, but you must take care of yourself. It sounds so simple, but many people spend more time maintaining their car than they do their bodies. Just like your car, your body needs to be properly fueled to run efficiently and properly maintained to look and feel its best.

THE MIND-BODY RELATIONSHIP

But there is much more to taking care of your health than just exercising your body. Modern living subjects you to constant stress, and there is often little time to devote to your physical and emotional well-being. You may not eat the right foods, take the right vitamins, or take the time to truly relax. The result can be a breakdown in your body's ability to stay well.

Each one of these areas of neglect can have a profound effect on your health. You are a beautiful, complex being made up of interconnected systems of physical and emotional energies. Your mental state affects your physical health, and your physical health affects your state of mind. And what you eat affects both. One can't be separated from the others.

This means that just taking vitamins, or just exercising, or just dieting, or just meditating will not make you healthy or bring you dynamic energy. In order to successfully maintain your health, you must maintain all three of your energies simultaneously. This is where TriEnergetics comes in. From the moment you start our program, you'll be balancing your physical, emotional, and mental energies.

YOU NEED A FOUNDATION, WALLS, AND A ROOF

Think of yourself as a beautiful building: a skyscraper, a cathedral, or a country home. In order to function, that building needs a stable foundation, strong supporting walls, and on top of it all, a roof for protection from the elements. If one is missing, the building will be incomplete. You can't have a roof without walls, and you can't have walls without a foundation. Each component works in concert with the others to achieve its goal.

Now relate this to your health. Nutrition forms the foundation upon which your health is built. Exercise gives you the strength to support your everyday activities, and meditation shelters your mind from the constant bombardment of stress that accompanies modern life.

YOU'LL BE AMAZED AT HOW EASY IT IS

We've made it easy to bring your body, mind, and nourishment into balance. All you need to do is take a little bit of time each day to follow the suggestions for that week.

In one easy-to-follow plan, you will get

› a complete, progressive fitness routine

› a comprehensive nutritional plan

› stress reduction techniques that include meditation, diaphragmatic breathing, and relaxation

› a complete nutritional supplementation plan

Our plan achieves results through a series of gentle, progressive changes. From the moment you start week one, you will make incremental changes in how you exercise, eat, and relax. Each change might not seem like much, but it builds upon the changes you made the week before. By the end of the six-week program, each of those small changes will have compounded. The result will be a quantum improvement in the way you look and feel.

IT'S TIME TO CHANGE

Modern society, especially in America, has strayed from wellness into sickness. The results are the many mental and physical health problems that plague us. The 2003 World Health Organization report showed that despite the United States' affluence and top-quality medical care, we rank twentieth in the world in average life expectancy. And it gets worse. The United States ranked twenty-third of all nations in average number of years lived in good health.

Is this good enough for you? It's not for us. We think this country needs a major health remedy. This remedy requires you to make a change. Making a change requires making a commitment. Do you have the motivation and the determination to make this change?

Moving On

Why not make good health your priority today? The first step toward wellness may be more difficult than the first step you took when you learned to walk, but the rewards will be worth it. It may be difficult to change a lifetime of attitudes, habits, and patterns, but it can be done. You can create a new you, the you that you would like to be.

Today is the perfect time for a new beginning. So let's move on and see how you can do this.

chapter 2

How to Use This Book:
Wellness Made Easy

We want to make it as easy as possible for you to get your health back on track. To help you get started, we've divided the book into two easy-to-read sections:

Fuel for Motivation. In chapters 3 through 9, you'll find the science behind the program. Here you can learn the principles of exercise, nutrition, and antioxidants. You'll learn about the deadly physiology of stress and the techniques you can use to combat it. You'll learn everything you need to fire your enthusiasm and get you ready to move forward on the path to better health. We'd like you to think of the "Fuel for Motivation" section as your own portable doctor, exercise physiologist, psychologist, meditation master, and nutritionist all combined in one place. These experts are at your disposal whenever you have questions about your health.

The TriEnergetics Program. In the remaining chapters, you'll find the nuts and bolts of the TriEnergetics program. We've divided the program into six weekly sessions. In each session, you'll find the goals that we'll ask you to attain for that week. These will include the small changes we want you to make in your nourishment, your exercise regimen, and your level of relaxation. With each week of the program, we'll give you all the information you'll need to progress smoothly and easily through that week.

GETTING STARTED

You don't need to read all of the "Fuel for Motivation" section before you get started on the TriEnergetics program. In fact, we encourage you to start right away. There's no reason to delay. Everything you'll need to understand each week's assignments is outlined for you in that week's chapter.

An ideal way to use this book would be to read the first few chapters in the "Fuel for Motivation" section, then complete the questionnaires at the beginning of the "TriEnergetics Program" section, and then launch into the program.

INTEGRATING YOUR BODY, MIND, AND NOURISHMENT

The goal of the TriEnergetics program is to help you integrate the three natural energies of your life: your body, your mind, and your nourishment. To this end, we've structured the TriEnergetics program to focus on each of these vital energies, individually and simultaneously.

Throughout this book, you will find a symbol being used to represent one of these key energies.

 Our symbol for body energy. This comes from the Taoist word *shen*. It literally means "body," "personal," or "one's whole life." The body is the firm foundation for the mind.

 Our symbol for mind energy. This comes from the Taoist word *jue*. It literally means "to perceive" or "to feel." The top half of this symbol means "to learn," while the bottom half means "to awaken." To become aware of the mind is to become aware of the spirit.

Our symbol for nourishment energy. This comes from the Taoist word *shi*. It literally means "to eat" or "food." Without controlling how you eat, you have no control over your life.

KEEP A JOURNAL OF YOUR JOURNEY

Throughout this book, we will present questionnaires, surveys, self-tests, and written exercises. We've found these to be extremely powerful in helping you to focus on your individual health needs. We've included space for you to write your answers right in this book. We want you to think of this book as the journal of your journey to better health and wellness.

Most importantly, during each week of the program, we'll present you with a weekly action plan. These self-tests will help motivate you to make positive changes in your life. To get the most from the program, take the time to think about the questions carefully and write your answers in the book.

Simply thinking about the questions isn't enough. The very act of writing will help to cement ideas and notions that you need to change. Don't shortchange your progress by ignoring this important part of the program.

ONE FINAL NOTE

This book is truly a collaborative effort of both of the authors, father and son, combining our many years of medical, exercise, and nutritional training; antioxidant research; and holistic and meditative practices. In writing, however, we found it cumbersome to relate individual experiences and anecdotes while maintaining the narrative of both authors.

In order to avoid confusion, we've created "Sandy's Stories" and "Todd's Tales" to allow each author to relate his own personal experience and anecdotes. We hope you'll find these experiences enlightening, insightful, and humorous.

Moving On

Now let's get started on the program and see the amazing results that await you.

PART I

Fuel for Motivation

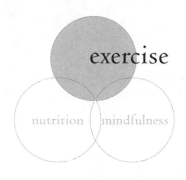

exercise

nutrition   mindfulness

chapter 3

Exercise Is the World's Best Medicine: The Secret That Everyone Already Knows

What if we were to tell you that we could write a prescription for you that would make you feel better, curb your appetite, help you lose weight, reduce stress and anxiety, help you sleep better, improve your self-image, increase your confidence, increase your sex drive, decrease your risk of having a heart attack or developing cancer, and slow down every aspect of the aging process?

Too good to be true, you might say. *Nothing can do all that.* We understand this kind of skepticism because we hear it all the time. But the truth is, such a magic elixir does exist. It is something that you can do every day, starting right now, to maximize your health and well-being. In fact, this magic elixir will do more than any fad diet, herbal remedy, or any other single health aid to improve your overall sense of wellness.

What is this magic elixir? It's exercise.

> If exercise could be packaged into a pill, it would be the single most prescribed and beneficial medicine in the nation.
>
> —Robert N. Butler

THE MAGIC ELIXIR

Exercise is a cornerstone of the TriEnergetics program. Not painful, burning exercise, but easy, progressive exercise that strengthens your muscles and your heart. Our exercise routines are designed specifically to give you all the benefits we've just mentioned. These exercises will make you look better and feel younger. And best of all, the exercises are fun to do.

That's saying a lot, isn't it? But the benefits of exercise have been documented time and time again by solid scientific research. What's more, the results are even better when the exercise program is incorporated into a comprehensive lifestyle program like TriEnergetics.

The TriEnergetics exercise plan will

› make you feel better

› curb your appetite

› help you lose weight

› reduce your stress and anxiety

› help you sleep better

› improve your cardiovascular fitness

› increase your lung capacity

› lower your cholesterol

› lower your blood pressure

› give you more energy

› reduce muscle fatigue

› strengthen your bones and joints

› improve your self-image

› increase your confidence

› increase your sex drive

› decrease your risk of having a heart attack

› decrease your risk of developing cancer

› slow down aging

YOU KNOW THIS, BUT DO YOU DO IT?

If you don't exercise regularly because you haven't wanted to or you haven't been motivated enough, you're not alone. Most Americans don't get enough exercise. The surgeon general of the United States has even spoken strongly of the need for exercise, but still people resist.

This problem is further compounded by contradictory statements made in popular health books. One noted health authority went so far as to say, "Whenever I go to a health club or gym and see people working out with pained expressions on their faces, I find myself thinking, if they are going to be expending that much energy with so little enjoyment, they might as well be doing something more useful—or at least more fun." Statements like this make us shudder. We know that there are people who will take this statement seriously and use it as justification for not moving off of the couch.

Let us state as clearly as possible: Exercise can and should be fun. If you are not enjoying your exercise and not feeling better because of it, then you are not exercising properly and may be harming yourself. That's not the way exercise should be.

A NEW PICTURE OF EXERCISE

Let's take a different view of exercise. Picture yourself enjoying moving your body in ways that make you feel good and light and energetic, and picture the changes in your body as your tummy begins to tighten and the love handles begin to trim and your muscles begin to harden.

That's a nicer picture, isn't it? And it's a realistic one as well. Our exercise routines will work wonders for your body, and you will actually have fun doing them. You'll see that effective exercise doesn't need to be painful or difficult. You'll be astounded at the progress you can make by just going with the natural energy flow of your body.

So let's shift into high gear. We want to get you as excited about exercise as we are. Then we'll give you a plan for incorporating it into your life.

Sandy's Story: Dad's Day at the Gym

I want to share a very personal story that involves my father and Todd's grandfather, Leo. He was a typical successful businessman, working long hours and eating big lunches. He made ample money and his life was good, but still he felt bad. Although he was only slightly overweight, most of his fat was stored in a spare tire around his waist. His arms and legs were thin. He had no energy, and when the workday was over, it was all he could do to come home, have dinner, and fall asleep in front of the TV.

Does this sound familiar?

Some years ago, I took a job filling in for a family practitioner in a little town in Missouri. Even in those days, I was a believer in regular exercise, and I spent my spare time helping the coaches at the local high school improve the conditioning of the students.

One day, my folks came to visit, to see their doctor son at work. You might say that my dad wanted to see how his investment in my education was paying off. Dad came to the high school while I was working with a group of students. He was curious about the exercise program and began to ask questions. I was astonished because I'd tried to get him to exercise before, but to no avail. I told him that the program was carefully thought out and that anyone of any age could begin and progress at their own pace. Dad listened, then asked if he could have one of the exercise books. I gladly gave it to him.

I next saw my dad six months later. His first words when he picked me up at the airport weren't "Hello" or "How are you doing?" His very first words were, "Hi, Sandy. Hit me in the stomach." You wouldn't believe the big smile on his face. His potbelly was gone, completely disappeared, and was he ever proud of himself.

I learned that his entire life had been transformed. He no longer fell asleep exhausted in front of the television. He had boundless energy and was taking a night class in Italian. Before, he had no time to exercise. Now he carried a gym bag wherever he went and exercised every day at noon at the health club or the local YMCA. He made friends wherever he went. His enthusiasm was contagious.

Needless to say, I didn't hit him in the stomach. I hugged him because I loved him and was proud of what he had accomplished.

• Todd's Tale: The Racquetball Grandpa

I wasn't around to see this amazing transformation in my grandfather. All of my memories of my grandfather are of a dynamic, energetic man who loved to go to the gym and work out, and crack jokes, and who—at the age of sixty-five—repeatedly gave me a trouncing on the racquetball court.

We could end the chapter with this story. It tells it all, describing an incredible transformation in a person's life. But we promised you some science, so read on.

THE HEART AT RISK

A tremendous amount is known about the effects of exercise on the mind and body. The most exciting research is in the relationship of physical activity and heart disease.

> Epidemiological studies have left no doubt as to the existence of a strong inverse relationship between physical exercise and coronary heart disease risk. The questions we need to address are not whether exercise is a real element for cardiovascular health, but what kind of exercise is needed, and how much, i.e., with what frequency, intensity, timing, and duration.
>
> —Ralph Paffenbarger

Heart disease is the leading killer in the United States, accounting for about 35 percent of all deaths. Heart disease is not a single illness but a general term for many different diseases of the heart and its vessels. Coronary artery disease is the major form of heart disease and is the single leading cause of death in the United States.

There are a number of risk factors that increase the probability of heart disease:

- male sex
- family history of heart disease

17

- history of stroke

- smoking

- type A personality

- high blood pressure

- high total cholesterol

- low level of high density lipoprotein cholesterol

- diabetes

- severe obesity

Obviously, you can't do anything about your family history or your sex, or whether you've had a stroke in the past, but you can affect all of the other risk factors. Let's look at them, one risk factor at a time.

SMOKING

Smoking is so harmful and incompatible with wellness that a discussion of smoking can be very brief. *Do not smoke.* If you are a smoker, quit. If you are not a smoker, don't start.

Now that that's out of the way, let's take a closer look at the other risk factors and see how exercise can give you control over each one of them.

TYPE A PERSONALITY

According to a study published in the *Journal of the American Medical Association* (Rosenman et al. 1975), the classic type A personality—competitive, impatient, uptight—is a heart attack waiting to happen. And that heart attack will likely happen sooner rather than later. In this study, researchers looked at 3,154 men between thirty-nine and fifty-nine years old. Each one of these guys was classified as having type A personality or not. The men were examined for heart disease about every five years.

In the first eight and a half years, 8 percent of the men developed heart disease. Those men with the strongest type A scores were twice as likely to have heart attacks as the calmer type B men.

Exercise has been shown to calm the harmful effects of the type A personality by reducing tension, anger, and anxiety (Jin 1989).

HIGH BLOOD PRESSURE

Fifteen to twenty percent of the adult American population, roughly fifty-eight million people, suffer from high blood pressure. This disease accounts for one of every four primary care visits and is the most common diagnosis for prescription management. High blood pressure (also known as *hypertension*) is a major risk factor for coronary heart disease, equivalent to smoking or high cholesterol.

The conventional method of treating hypertension is with medication. More than ten million hypertensive patients in this country spend $2.5 billion annually on high blood pressure medicines. This far exceeds the amount spent on any other disease.

Exercise Lowers Blood Pressure

There are alternatives to medication for the treatment of hypertension. A good number of people with high blood pressure can be helped or even cured with exercise.

Paffenbarger and Lee (1997) studied 15,000 male Harvard alumni and found that those who did not engage in vigorous sports or other activity were at a 35 percent greater risk of developing hypertension than those who did. They also showed that even in those men who had hypertension, exercise reduced their blood pressure.

HIGH TOTAL CHOLESTEROL

The body naturally synthesizes cholesterol, which is needed to form cell membranes and is found in abundance in brain and nerve tissue. Excess cholesterol can't be put to good use and unfortunately gets deposited in places where you don't want it, such as in the lining of blood vessels, where it blocks circulation.

Cholesterol and other fats are transported through the blood by particles called *lipoproteins*. There are three major lipoproteins in the blood: *high density lipoprotein* (HDL), *low density lipoprotein* (LDL), and *very low density lipoprotein* (VLDL). The HDL particle acts as a cholesterol shuttle, taking it from the blood and body cells to the liver, where it's disposed of.

LDLs, on the other hand, are often called the bad lipoproteins (or bad cholesterol) because they take their cholesterol to various body cells, where it's deposited. Some of this cholesterol is used by the tissues to build cells, and some is returned to the liver. LDL is the major cholesterol carrier in the body.

When excessively high, LDLs contribute to the development of *atherosclerosis* (thickening and hardening of the arteries). LDLs stick to the walls of the arteries, including those that supply blood to the heart. A high level of LDL (160 mg/dL and above) causes an increased risk of heart disease.

If serum cholesterol levels are lowered, the incidence of coronary artery disease decreases. Reducing plasma cholesterol levels by only 25 percent can reduce coronary artery disease by as much as 50 percent. An optimal level of LDL cholesterol is less than 100 mg/dL.

LOW LEVELS OF HIGH DENSITY LIPOPROTEIN CHOLESTEROL

HDLs are often called the good cholesterol. Some experts think that HDLs help keep the blood vessels clean by removing excess cholesterol buildup. According to the American Heart Association, a high level of HDL cholesterol may protect against heart attack. People with a low level of HDL (less than 40 mg/dL) have a higher risk of heart attack. It's good to have your HDL above 60 mg/dL to really help protect your heart.

According to the National Institute of Health, in order to reduce the possibility of developing coronary heart disease, your total cholesterol should be less than 200 mg/dL.

Exercise Regulates Cholesterol

Exercise has a powerful, beneficial effect on serum cholesterol. Men and women who participate in vigorous exercise have lower levels of bad cholesterol and higher levels of good cholesterol. In fact, one study in the *New England Journal of Medicine* showed that even changing your diet won't effectively lower LDL cholesterol unless you exercise as well.

Regular exercise not only helps prevent heart disease, it's also the cornerstone of cardiac rehabilitation after a heart attack or after coronary bypass surgery. Patients recovering from a heart attack begin a gentle exercise program within twenty-four hours and are advised to continue it if they want to stay healthy.

DIABETES

Having diabetes seriously increases your risk of getting coronary artery disease. According to the American Heart Association, even if your blood sugar levels are under control, simply having diabetes will increase your chance of having a heart attack. In fact, about 75 percent of all diabetics die from some form of vascular disease. If you have diabetes, it is critically important that you manage your sugar levels well and monitor your blood sugar regularly. Exercise is a critical component of diabetes management because it helps you to decrease blood glucose levels and increase the efficacy of insulin (Wu 2005).

SEVERE OBESITY

Americans are among the fattest people in the world. There are over 34 million obese adults in the United States carrying an excess of 2.3 billion pounds of fat. Compounding this problem is the fact that Americans are still getting fatter. Despite the increased public awareness of the health risks of obesity, the number of obese people in America has increased by 50 percent since 1998. In the South Atlantic states, the number of obese people rose by 67 percent. In Georgia alone, the number of obese people skyrocketed 102 percent.

Why is this so important? Because being overweight can kill you. An increased risk of heart disease is just one of the problems that plague those who are overweight. Other problems include

- increased incidence of hypertension

- increased LDL cholesterol levels

- increased incidence of diabetes

- increased incidence of cancer

- increased incidence of sudden death

You don't need to be skinny to be healthy, but there are definite health risks in being overweight.

Why is there so much obesity in one of the most prosperous nations in the world? Blame it on lifestyle, blame it on bad eating, and most importantly, blame it on not enough exercise.

Exercise Will Help You Lose Weight

A fabulous study from Boston University Medical Center showed clearly the effects of exercise on weight loss. They put 110 overweight cops and other city employees on a strict diet. Half were placed in a supervised exercise program, ninety minutes of exercise three times a week. The other half were instructed to not change their exercise habits.

After eight weeks, the dieters had lost an average of twenty-three pounds; those who were both dieting and exercising had lost twenty-seven pounds. The difference isn't that impressive, but eighteen months after the study ended, the diet-only participants gained back more than 90 percent of the weight they'd lost. The diet-and-exercise folks who continued to exercise didn't gain back a single pound! That's because the exercise helped the dieters to maintain a more effective metabolism for weight control.

And there's more. Many people feel that they have a genetic predisposition to being overweight, and no matter what they try, they will remain heavy. Well, we've got good news for you. A major English and Australian study published in the *Annals of Internal Medicine* (Weinsier 1999) found that exercise had a greater impact on weight than diet or any other factor, including genes. Another study (Samaras et al. 1999) looked at identical twins who grew up in the same household. They found that the single most important factor in determining any weight difference between the twins was the amount of exercise they performed.

If You Want to Lose Weight, You've Got to Move Your Behind

Why is exercise so important for sustained weight loss? The answer is simple. It's based on how much energy your body uses each day.

The average 154-pound male needs about 1,600 calories a day to maintain his normal body functions. This is his *basal metabolic rate,* or BMR. If this average person was inactive physically and used only another 300 to 800 calories a day on physical activity, he would require about 1,900 to 2,400 calories a day to maintain his body. Anything he ate over this amount would be converted to fat.

Top athletes, on the other hand, frequently match their basal metabolic energy expenditure through intense exercise. A very active average female could easily burn an additional 1,000 to 1,600 calories a day because of her physical activity.

Calculate Your Basal Energy Expenditure

To get an idea of what your own basal metabolic rate is, use the following formula:

For males: $BMR = 66 + 13.8(W) + 5(H) - 6.8(A)$

For females: $BMR = 655 + 9.6(W) + 1.8(H) - 4.7(A)$

BMR = calories per day

W = current weight in kilograms (1 kilogram = 2.2 pounds)

H = height in centimeters (1 inch = 2.54 centimeters)

A = age in years

Let's look at an example. Say a forty-five-year-old woman wants to know her daily basal expenditure of calories. She is five feet, six inches tall and weighs 140 pounds. Using this formula, you can see that

W = 140 pounds ÷ 2.2 kilograms per pound = 64 kilograms

H = five feet, six inches × twelve inches per foot = 66 inches; 66 inches × 2.54 centimeters per inch = 168 centimeters

A = 47 years

So $BMR = 655 + 9.6(64) + 1.8(168) - 4.7(47)$

$BMR = 655 + 614 + 302 - 221$

$BMR = 1,350$ calories

23

This is the amount of energy that she expends each and every day just to keep her body functioning. If she's relatively inactive, anything she eats over this will most likely be stored as fat. If she exercises regularly, she'll burn even more calories than this.

Create Metabolically Active Muscle

The other benefit of exercise for weight loss is that as you exercise, you build up more muscle mass and get rid of fat. Muscle has a very active metabolism. Fat has a very slow metabolic rate. The more you exercise, the more muscle you build. The greater your muscle mass, the higher your basic metabolic rate and the more calories you will burn every single day.

THE FOUNTAIN OF YOUTH

Exercise not only helps you lose weight and fight disease, it will also help to keep you young and vital.

So, what does it mean to get older? George Burns wrote, "You'll know when you are old when everything hurts and what doesn't hurt doesn't work; when you get winded playing chess; when you stoop to tie your shoelaces and ask yourself what else you can do while you are down there." Do you think that this applies to everyone? Does aging mean that your body must deteriorate?

When we were in medical school, we were taught that as people got older, they developed chronic diseases, lost their strength, lost their physical fitness, and developed soft bones. Who wants to look forward to such misery? Not us, and probably not you.

But did you know that most of these changes are exactly what astronauts experienced when they were inactive during prolonged periods of weightlessness? The absence of gravity caused weakness, bone resorption, and a loss of physical fitness. When a program of regular exercise was added to all space missions, these problems reduced significantly. Similarly, much of the deterioration attributed to aging can be explained not by the fact that people are getting older but by the fact that they are exercising less and less as they age.

You will age. That is a fact of life. But you can age in a way that creates a healthy, active life for you. A balanced, sensible program of exercise will help you stay younger and healthier. Exercise is probably the only true fountain of youth.

BEEF UP YOUR BONES

Just as astronauts lose bone density during periods of inactivity in space, inactive older people—particularly postmenopausal women—lose bone density. Ten million Americans over the age of fifty have osteoporosis, while another 34 million are at risk. Some of them become deformed, with big humps on their backs, and most of them suffer considerable pain. According to the 2004 report issued by the surgeon general, each year about 1.5 million people suffer a bone fracture related to osteoporosis.

Hormones and genetics account for some of the problem, but inactivity is the major culprit. People lose bone mass rapidly when muscular stress on the legs is reduced. A person confined to bed can lose an average of 1 percent of his bone mineral content per week.

EXERCISE YOUR BONES

Exercise contributes to the development of strong bones.

Thirty elderly women, average age eighty-one, were studied for bone loss. Half participated in a forty-minute exercise program three times a week. The other half had no formal exercise. The sedentary group had a bone mineral content loss of 3.28 percent during the thirty-six months of the study, while the physically active group had a 2.29 percent *gain.*

In another study (Smith et al. 1984), women aged thirty-five to sixty-five who exercised vigorously for forty-five minutes three times weekly for three to four years increased their bone mineral mass almost 3 percent. This compared to a 2.4 percent loss per year for a matched sedentary group.

If you want healthy, strong bones, get yourself started on a progressive exercise routine.

STAY HEALTHY, STAY YOUNG

Exercise is not only for the young. Countless people have completely revitalized their lives through exercise.

- ### Amazing Mavis

Mavis Lindgren has been called "Amazing Mavis" by Sports Illustrated. *As a child, she suffered with pneumonia, and annual bouts of severe bronchitis dogged her throughout her adulthood. She did not start exercising until she was in her early sixties and was twenty pounds overweight.*

She began walking faithfully every day and slowly increased her walking distance. As her strength improved, she began to jog. Her health gradually improved, and she found that she loved to jog. So she began running. At age seventy, she was running five miles six times a week. Her son, a doctor of medicine, urged her to train for marathon running, so she doubled her mileage.

Between ages seventy and eighty-one, she raced in fifty-two marathons, breaking her own age-group world record four different times. Amazing!

Of course, you don't have to become a marathon runner to achieve wellness. We take great pride in the number of people who come to our programs tired, stressed, and overweight and leave with a more positive, energetic mind and body.

- ### Bart's Recovery

Bart is just such an example. For years, he'd suffered from stiffness and soreness in his back and hips, and as a result, he felt frustrated and depressed. He hadn't exercised in years for fear of aggravating his ailing back. Consequently, he gained more than sixty pounds. As he gained more weight, he became more depressed and began eating uncontrollably. Bart's blood pressure sailed out of control as his body continued to deteriorate. Finally, at the age of thirty-five, Bart came face-to-face with his own mortality: he suffered a heart attack. By the time we met him, Bart was at his wit's end.

But all that changed. Within six weeks after starting the TriEnergetics program, Bart had learned how to control his eating. He gave up junk food and kept a handy supply of healthy snacks with him at all times. Starting the exercise program slowly, he quickly progressed to the point that he easily walked several miles a day. In fact, he learned to enjoy walking so much, he purchased a treadmill so he could walk on rainy days. With the aid of the stress management techniques, Bart learned how to handle his stress and battle his depression, and he gained a new enthusiasm for life.

Bart was so excited by his improved energy and motivated by his renewed confidence, he went on to become the leader for a local men's group. Bart's life was completely transformed.

Success comes in all sizes and shapes. We want you to find the success that's waiting for you.

A SOUND MIND IN A SOUND BODY

As we said in the beginning, each aspect of your body's natural energy—your physical, mental, and nourishment energies—exist in concert with every other aspect of your body. What affects one affects the others. It should come as no surprise, then, that in addition to its numerous beneficial effects on the body, exercise also improves your emotional state.

Exercise has been shown to help alleviate mental anxiety and depression and burn off stress. It quiets the mind.

The amazing, calming effects of exercise have been known for years. The ancient Greeks maintained that exercise made the mind more lucid. John F. Kennedy echoed this Greek ideal when he said, "Physical fitness is not only one of the most important keys to a healthy body, it is the basis of dynamic and creative intellectual activity. Hardy spirits and tough minds usually inhabit sound bodies."

The ancient Taoist sage Sun Ssu-mo also recognized this fact. He stated that in order to nurture calmness of the mind, a person must keep himself as fluid and flexible as possible. "When the body doesn't move," Sun Ssu-mo said, "essence cannot flow, and when essence cannot flow, energy becomes stagnant."

Modern science has confirmed Sun Ssu-mo's beliefs.

Exercise produces endorphins. *Endorphins* are morphinelike chemicals produced by the body. During exercise, the pituitary increases production of endorphins. These endorphins race through the blood to the brain and cause a feeling of euphoria. They also change the electrical activity of the brain, increasing the emission of alpha waves. These alpha waves have been shown by psychological research to be associated with relaxed, meditative states.

Exercise enhances neurotransmitter activity in the brain. *Neurotransmitters,* such as norepinephrine, dopamine, and serotonin, are compounds that serve as chemical messengers in the brain. They elevate mood and counter depression.

People who exercise regularly feel better because they look better. They look better because exercise helps them control their weight and firm up their muscle tone. As the saying goes, as you look, so you will feel.

THE ROAD TO IMMORTALITY?

No one can guarantee that you will live longer if you exercise, but it sure looks promising. Paffenbarger and Lee (1997) showed that Harvard alumni whose energy output in active exercise totaled at least 2,000 calories a week experienced a 28 percent reduction in all causes of death. Those who expended 3,500 calories a week in exercise had a death rate that was 50 percent lower. Life expectancy was more than two years greater for those who expended more than 2,000 calories a week exercising, compared with those who expended less than 500 calories a week.

Eight great health benefits of TriEnergetics exercise

> reduced risk of heart disease   > increased muscle tone

> lowered blood pressure   > increased bone density

> lowered LDL cholesterol   > calmer mind

> weight loss   > longer life

KNOW YOUR LIMITS

As we've said, you don't have to be a marathon runner or fitness fanatic to get all of the wonderful benefits of exercise. You do have to move your body, though, in a way that is sufficient to increase your heart rate and stretch your muscles.

One mistake many people make when they first start exercising is that they overdo it. We see this every year at the local fitness club. Come January, the club is packed with new members, each of whom has made the New Year's resolution to finally get off the couch and get in shape. While the goal is admirable, the way they go about it is wrong.

The first Monday of each year, the warriors race into the club, work out at a feverish intensity, shower up, and go home. They feel great that day, but come the morning they can barely get out of bed. Every muscle is sore. The following day they're still sore, so they skip their workout that day—and the next, and the next. Soon they're back on the couch, where they were before.

You have to know your limits. When it comes to exercise, you have to move your body at an intensity that is beneficial for you, but it does you no good to overdo it.

● Sandy's Story: Running with the Astronauts

I learned this lesson myself one day when I went running with the astronauts. Let me explain. After my internship in internal medicine, I joined the Air Force and became a member of the faculty of the School of Aviation Medicine. I had a number of interesting assignments there, but without a doubt, my most interesting assignment was as part of the medical team that evaluated the mental and physical health of the astronaut candidates for the space program, Project Gemini. Needless to say, all of the candidates were very intelligent and courageous. I learned the hard way that they were also in incredible physical condition.

My lesson began when one of the candidates asked if there was a handball court on the base and whether he and a buddy could get a game. I smiled. Not only was there a handball court nearby, but several of us doctors played every noon, and some of us were very good. We also ran every day before we played. We prided ourselves in being in top physical shape.

I figured that I'd teach this test pilot a lesson in humility, so I told him that we played a little handball and we'd enjoy playing a match. I also mentioned that we usually jogged a little bit to warm up before we played. I didn't tell him that the jog was really a three-mile run along the flight line of Brooks Air Force Base in 110-degree heat.

The next day, the two astronaut candidates met us at noon for the jog and the handball game. During the jog, my group ran as fast as we could, really pushing our bodies, trying to beat our guests into submission. But it didn't work that way. At the two-mile mark, one of the candidates said, "Doc, it's just too hot out here to be running like this. If you'll excuse us, we'll meet you at the handball court."

And with that, they just took off and sprinted to the gym, leaving us in their dust, our jaws hanging open with amazement. We forced ourselves to finish the run. Twenty minutes later, they promptly whipped us on the handball court.

I never ran with an astronaut again.

EXERCISE THE TRIENERGETICS WAY

Exercise doesn't have to be painful, grueling, dirty, or sweaty to be beneficial. You don't have to run with the astronauts or get your body too sore to move off the couch. You can get all the benefits of exercise in a way that is easy and—best of all—fun. In fact, the cornerstone of the TriEnergetics aerobic exercise program is a relaxing, pleasant activity you can do any time of the day, with a friend or loved one, and it doesn't require any extra equipment or a health club membership.

We're talking about walking.

WALK YOUR WAY TO HEALTH

Walking at a good pace burns as many calories as running, is easy on the joints, and can be a fun way to get in shape. What could be nicer than walking through a park with a companion, enjoying the fresh air and watching the sunset?

Perhaps you think you really need to pound your body in order to get effective exercise. This simply isn't true. The health benefits of walking vigorously (faster than a stroll, but slower than running) are many and have been supported by sound clinical science.

Here are five great reasons to walk for your health.

You'll live longer. A recent study in the *New England Journal of Medicine* (Manson et al. 2002) showed that women who walked briskly at least three hours per week reduced their risk of heart attack by 30 to 40 percent. Another study from the Honolulu Heart Program (Kagan 1996) found that adults who walked an average of two miles a day reduced their risk of premature death by 50 percent.

You'll burn more calories. Walking burns more calories than riding on a stationary bike. Researchers at the Medical College of Wisconsin found that walking on a treadmill burned more calories than exercising with any other indoor machine (Fitness Fact 1998).

You'll lose weight. Not only does exercise burn calories to help you lose weight, but as you exercise over time and increase muscle mass, your body's metabolism speeds up and you will burn more calories.

You'll build stronger bones. Walking and other weight-bearing exercises promote bone growth. Not only that, walking can relieve pain in your lower back. In fact, the best thing you can do for chronic low back pain is to perform moderate, low-impact exercise, like walking, three times a week.

You'll sleep better. The Stanford Exercise and Sleep Study showed that when men and women with insomnia walk briskly thirty to forty minutes four times a week, they fall asleep faster at night and sleep for nearly an hour longer.

Moving On

There are no pills you can purchase or elixir you can drink that will do as much for you as a systematic program of regular, progressive exercise, like the TriEnergetics program.

In the next chapter, we will introduce another key component in keeping the body supple, energetic, and agile: how you nourish your body.

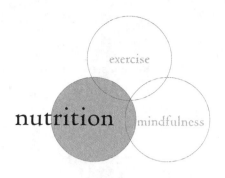

exercise

nutrition *mindfulness*

chapter 4

Why Diets Don't Work: Understanding How Your Body Uses Food

Let's talk about food. It's the basic building blocks of life. The fuel in your engine. The raw materials for the construction of your body. Yet there is more confusion about how to eat than any other aspect of health. You'd think that after all the years experts have spent studying nutritional science and biochemistry, Americans would finally understand what a healthy, energizing diet is.

But the truth is that most people still don't know. Instead, the mass media focuses on the latest fad diet: high protein and low fat this day, low protein and high carb the next; low carb, high protein; moderate fat, moderate protein, high carb; complex carbs, simple sugars, no protein. No wonder people are confused.

Then it gets worse. The media tells us about the all-protein diet, the grapefruit diet, the cabbage soup diet, the all-bran diet, the starvation diet, the drink-my-product-and-look-gorgeous-tomorrow diet. It's enough to make your head swim.

The facts are really quite simple.

DIETS DON'T WORK

On any diet, you will lose weight temporarily—and it will all come back. This has been shown over and over again in rigorous scientific research. But most people still refuse to believe this. They think that the only way to lose weight or to be healthy is to force themselves onto a radical diet. They think that they have to starve the body so that they'll burn up the fat stores.

This is wrong. Food is not the enemy. You can't starve your body to lose fat or become healthy. That simply isn't the way the body works. Just as you can't run your car on an empty gas tank, you can't run your body without food.

You must feed your body the energy it needs to live—the energy it needs to replicate DNA and divide its cells and move its muscles and build its enzymes. If you eat properly, the proper foods and the proper combinations, you can eat just about as much as you want of whatever you want. The weight will come off and stay off naturally. You can actually eat more food and still lose weight.

In this chapter, we'll show you why the latest diet fad is doomed to fail. You'll learn how your body processes the food you eat, so you'll understand what your body really needs. We'll give you the lowdown on carbohydrates, fats, proteins, and fiber.

Then, in chapter 5, we'll introduce you to the TriEnergetics approach to eating, an approach that not only promotes your optimum weight but increases your energy, maximizes your vitality, and helps your body to naturally fight disease.

DIET MYTHS

Let's begin by taking a look at some common diet myths. A diet myth is a bit of misinformation that is packaged to convince you to accept it as the gospel truth. Diet myths are propagated by carefully crafted advertising campaigns as well as idle office talk.

The problem is, the myths aren't true. Believing in these myths can send you down the wrong road. Here's what the myths truly mean.

Seven Common Diet Myths

- When you diet, you lose weight.

- Diets are healthy.

- When you diet, you lose fat.

- It is harder to lose weight when you are older because your metabolism slows down.

- Your metabolism slows down when you diet because your body goes into a starvation mode.

- By simply reducing fat in your diet, you'll lose weight.

- Losing weight is simply a matter of watching what you eat.

Myth Number One: When You Diet, You Lose Weight.

Yes, you lose weight when you diet because you are restricting calories, but the weight loss is only temporary if you don't also make lifestyle changes. A staggering 98 percent of those who diet will gain the weight back. Exercise is the biggest factor in determining whether dieters gain the weight back. Those who exercise in addition to changing their diet are far more likely to keep the weight off. Dieting alone is not the answer.

Myth Number Two: Diets Are Healthy

Fad diets are like fashion trends: they come and go. They are sensationalized by their proponents and by the media, frequently without any clinical studies to support their health claims.

Be careful. Most fad diets are not healthy. Many are downright danger-ous. Some create conditions of acidosis, ketosis, or nitrogen imbalance. Others that advocate high fat intake can contribute to the development of heart disease or cancer.

The high-protein diet fiasco. The biggest contributor to this myth recently has been the high-protein, low-carbohydrate diet. Proponents claim that you will lose weight and be healthier on a diet high in animal protein and fat and low in carbohydrates. They claim that calories from fat or protein don't count as long as you don't eat carbohydrates.

Part of this claim is true. You will lose weight on the high-protein diet, mainly because as you cut out the carbohydrates, you cut out 99 percent of snack foods. Less snack food equals fewer calories, so you lose weight. You also won't feel hungry on this diet because it takes a long time to digest protein and fat, so you'll feel fuller longer.

But this doesn't mean that it's healthy. In fact, this may be one of the unhealthiest diets unleashed on the American public in some time.

Dangers of a diet too high in protein and fat. Here are some of the dangers inherent in a high-animal-protein, high-fat, low-carbohydrate diet.

- The high load of saturated, polyunsaturated, and trans fats can clog your arteries and promote heart disease. Although proponents claim that this diet doesn't increase serum cholesterol levels, there is very little scientific evidence to support this.

- High amounts of fat in your diet can cause a sharp increase in factor VII in your blood, leading to heart attacks. (We'll talk more about this later in the chapter.)

- The high protein load can have a dangerous effect on the kidneys.

- The ban on complex carbohydrates greatly diminishes the amount of fiber you eat.

- Numerous studies have linked a diet heavy in animal protein with an increased risk of cancers.

- Without carbohydrates in your diet, you don't burn fat completely, resulting in a buildup of waste products called *ketones. Ketosis,* the dangerous accumulation of ketones, causes nausea, headaches, dehydration, and weakness and can lead to gout and kidney stones.

- The low-carbohydrate diet requires that you cut out many fruits and vegetables because of their sugar content. This completely ignores the fact that more than two hundred studies have shown that fruits and vegetables reduce the risk of cancers of the lung, stomach, prostate, esophagus, cervix, endometrium, bladder, kidney, and breast. Produce is packed with nutrients, antioxidants, flavonoids, and fiber.

Seven Dangers of a High-Protein, High-Fat Diet

› clogged arteries

› increased factor VII, leading to heart attacks

› kidney damage

› deprivation of plant nutrients and antioxidants

› diminished fiber

› increased risk of cancers

› ketosis

There is nothing healthy about the high-protein diet.

Simply losing weight does not make you healthy. When it comes to evaluating fad diets, use your common sense.

Myth Number Three: When You Diet, You Lose Fat

The point of dieting is to lose fat, right? The fact is that when you diet, you lose muscle and keep the fat.

How can that be? After all, everyone has seen the horrible pictures of starving people who are only skin and bones. Haven't they lost all of their body fat? No, they have lost almost all of their muscle mass and only some of their fat.

When you starve yourself, your body is forced to feed upon itself to generate energy. Muscles are a ready source of energy, and they are consumed rapidly. Not the fat. The body holds on to fat to maintain a store of energy in case there is a prolonged period without adequate food. In the process of starvation, a little fat is lost with the muscle, but most of it is hoarded until the end.

So, what happens when you go on that special diet to create a new you? Perhaps you lose forty pounds initially. Then you quit dieting and begin to put on weight. Maybe you only gain thirty-five pounds back. That's progress, correct? After all, you are five pounds lighter.

Wrong again. You are probably fatter now than you were before. Even though you weigh five pounds less, you gained back fat and lost lean muscle, when you really wanted to gain muscle and lose fat.

No one goes on a diet to get fatter, but that is exactly what happens if you diet and don't exercise.

Myth Number Four: It Is Harder to Lose Weight When You Are Older Because Your Metabolism Slows Down

Your metabolism may slow down when you are older, but it is not slowing down *because* you are older. It is slowing down because you are fatter.

As people age, they tend to exercise less while eating as much as they did when they were younger. These excess calories have to go someplace, usually to the hips and middle. People who are inactive lose muscle mass and replace it with fat. Fat has a lower metabolic rate than muscle. Therefore, the more fat people have, the slower their metabolism becomes and the easier it is to get even fatter. This creates a vicious circle. As people get fatter, they tend to exercise even less, which makes them fatter still.

There is a gradual decrease in your basal metabolic rate as you age. This translates to a gradually increasing weight gain if you continue to eat the same amount of food. Let's look at the change in BMR for an average woman five feet, five inches tall and 121 pounds.

FEMALE BASAL METABOLIC RATE		
Age	BMR Calories	Pounds of Fat Gained per Year
20	1,382	0
40	1,363	2
50	1,325	6
60	1,267	12

For an average man five feet, ten inches tall and 155 pounds, the numbers are worse.

MALE BASAL METABOLIC RATE		
Age	BMR Calories	Pounds of Fat Gained per Year
20	1,736	0
40	1,649	5.8
50	1,627	8.2
60	1,593	11.8

As you age, you need to increase—not decrease—your physical activity to maintain a healthy, vital body and prevent the fat from accumulating.

Another metabolic problem occurs when people get older and stop exercising. Their muscles get lazy and forget how to burn fat. That means that when they do exercise, their muscles burn the glucose that is readily available; then their muscles start to ache and they have to stop exercising. This is part of being out of shape, and it is another reason why people who don't exercise have trouble losing fat. It takes regular exercise to train muscles to burn fat.

Myth Number Five: Your Metabolism Slows Down When You Diet Because Your Body Goes into a Starvation Mode

Yes, your metabolism slows down when you diet, but it's not because your body shuts down or goes into a starvation mode. Your body just doesn't work that way. Every cell in your body is metabolically active twenty-four hours a day, and the only time a cell shuts down is when it's dead. Your body is very alive, and its basic functions run around the clock.

What happens when you diet is that there is less food to be digested, and therefore fewer calories are used to process the food. Your basic energy requirements are decreased, and as a result, your basic metabolic rate slows down. The less you eat, the lower your basal metabolic rate and the fewer calories you need to maintain the necessary functions of your body. In other words, the less you eat, the fewer calories your body burns and the harder it becomes to lose weight.

In order to lose weight, you must exercise as you cut down on your eating. Exercise raises your metabolic rate and burns calories.

Myth Number Six: By Simply Reducing Fat in Your Diet, You'll Lose Weight

It's true that high-fat foods are also high-calorie foods, so by eliminating the fat, you will take in fewer calories. Combine this with a good exercise routine and a stress reduction program, and you will probably lose weight. But there is more to losing weight than simply cutting out the fat.

One of the biggest mistakes people commonly make is believing that low-fat foods are low in calories. This is not necessarily the case. Most processed low-fat foods substitute huge amounts of sugar to compensate for the flavor lost when the fat was removed. Low-fat foods are often packed with calories. Further, since many of these foods aren't as satisfying as their high-fat counterparts, you might be tempted to overindulge in the low-fat variety, taking in more calories than if you ate the high-fat version.

Myth Number Seven: Losing Weight Is Simply a Matter of Watching What You Eat

There is some truth to this myth. In order to lose weight, you must watch what you eat, taking care to avoid high-calorie, high-fat foods. But there is much more to weight loss than careful eating.

As we've said before, the body is a beautiful, complex creation, and all of your energies are interrelated. By now, you know that you need to exercise to lose weight, but there is even more to you than your physical being. There is also your mind.

Your mental energy can have a profound effect on how your body works, moves, and burns calories. To effectively control your weight, you must find mental peace and harmony. This is why the TriEnergetics approach to health integrates nutrition and exercise with mindfulness and stress reduction. In the next chapter, we'll show you how to integrate your mind and your eating.

THE BUSINESS OF FAT

It's no wonder so many people fall prey to these diet myths. Look around you. In America, we have everything in abundance. Lots of junk food, lots of greasy restaurants, lots of fast-food outlets—lots of ways to get fat.

Approximately 127 million adults in the United States are overweight, 60 million are obese, and 9 million are severely obese. Right now, 65 percent of U.S. adults age twenty and older are overweight, and 31 percent are obese.

A new study (Goel et al. 2004) found that obesity is relatively rare in people who've just moved to the United States. Only 8 percent of immigrants who had lived in the United States for less than one year were obese, but that number soared to 19 percent among those who'd been here for at least fifteen years. The American diet is so bad, it is an equal opportunity fattener.

The health of Americans is getting worse and worse. People are used to being tired all the time, drained of energy and vitality. They're used to chronic aches and pains, stomach and intestinal problems, high blood pressure, and heart disease. They're used to feeling awful.

This isn't just a cosmetic problem; it is killing people. In fact, a new study published in the *New England Journal of Medicine* (Olshansky et al. 2005) found that the obesity epidemic will cause U.S. life expectancy to dramatically decrease for the first time in centuries if Americans don't make major lifestyle changes.

OUR MOUTHS ARE AT THEIR MERCY

This isn't happening by chance. Americans are being programmed to eat improperly and to feel like garbage. Powerful megacorporations produce the overly processed, vitamin-depleted fast food, snack food, and junk food, and they want you to eat it. They use multimillion-dollar marketing budgets to cram images of fatty snacks into your subconscious with their endless stream of commercials and advertisements. You can't escape it.

You better believe that the marketing people know just how to get you to crave their products. They've spent billions of dollars studying consumer behavior. They know just what buttons to press to get you to run for that candy bar or doughnut or hamburger. The commercials show a hunk of a guy finishing a workout and reaching for a "satisfying" candy bar or a beautiful woman stepping into a bar and ordering a beer. They've made unhealthy eating a part of our culture.

DIETING IS BIG BUSINESS

The diet industry has become a $33 billion per year business, capitalizing on the national desire to lose weight. Diet companies sell their diets or gimmicks or powdered drinks and try to convince you that you will lose weight. As you know by now, these diets don't work.

It's one vicious, self-serving circle of bad foods and bad diets. That's just the way these industries want it. Believe us, these people are making a lot of money. They don't want you to lose weight. If you did, they'd lose their consumer pool. They want you fat.

DYING TO BE THIN

Any prescription pill that promises weight loss becomes an instant rage. During 1998 alone, fifty million prescriptions for fen-phen were written. People were so desperate to rid themselves of fat that they flocked to their doctor's offices and signed up for these "miracle" pills.

Fen-phen was a boon to the pharmaceutical industry and to a lot of unscrupulous doctors. Some doctors even prescribed the drugs over the Internet without ever seeing or examining the person. Just give them the money and they'd get you the pills.

As it turned out, these pills kill people.

IF YOU CAN'T LOSE IT, REMOVE IT

It is a sad comment on our society that liposuction and stomach stapling have become accepted methods of weight loss. *If you can't lose weight naturally*, the thinking goes, *just suck the fat out of your body!* We know many perfectly healthy people who have succumbed to the plastic surgery advertising barrage and gone under the knife. They've all said the same things:

I've dieted and dieted, and I just can't get the weight off.

I've tried exercising, but my love handles don't budge.

These fat areas are genetic. Nothing but surgery will get them off.

These people are just setting themselves up for another fall and making some slick plastic surgeon richer in the process. People can suck all the fat out of their bodies that they want, but unless they learn the basic principles of nutrition and exercise, that fat will just come right back.

Americans have been taught to believe that their weight is out of their control. People believe that they are victims. They think that the only way out of this cycle of obesity is to rely on a drug, a doctor—anything or anyone but themselves.

43

YOU HAVE THE POWER

Losing weight is more than just having a probe inserted into your abdomen and turning the suction on to high. Losing weight is more than jumping on the latest diet fad or swallowing toxic drugs.

You have the power to control your weight. You can take the control of your life away from the media, the food conglomerates, the diet industry, the plastic surgeons, and the drug companies.

KNOWLEDGE IS THE KEY

Losing weight comes naturally and easily when you incorporate the basics of good nutrition with a holistic lifestyle program of exercise, nutritional supplementation, and relaxation. You can learn how to eat right and how to move your body to burn fat and strengthen your heart. You can learn how to balance your diet with supplements to ward off aging changes, and you can learn how to control the stress in your life in a way that maximizes your feeling of well-being and helps prevent disease.

It's really quite simple. We're not selling a diet. We don't want you fat. We want to teach you a complete lifestyle strategy that will make you the ruler of your own body. We want to give you the tools to feel younger and look better. And all of that starts with eating.

YOU ARE WHAT YOU EAT

Proper eating is essential for your health. You must take in enough calories to supply your body with life-giving energy. You must take in proteins and carbohydrates and fats to live. How you do this, and in what quantities, is very important. Improper eating not only robs you of energy and causes you to get fat, but it also causes disease.

You don't have to have a master's degree in biochemistry to understand the principles of nutrition. You just need to know what food really is and how that food is converted by your body into usable energy.

UNDERSTANDING YOUR BODY

What we're going to talk about is your body's natural metabolism. This is what you need to understand to burn fat, build muscle, and feel dynamically better. As you will see, these are not rules carved in stone. But you need to be aware of your body, your health, and your exercise level to understand what you should be eating.

The word "metabolism" comes from the Greek *metabolos,* which means changeable. The science of metabolism deals with how the body changes that steak or piece of pie into simple chemicals that are transported in your blood to your cells, where they are used to build new proteins and enzymes and to provide energy for replicating your DNA and moving chemicals into and out of your cells. Here are the basic concepts of metabolism.

Every cell in your body is a miniature chemical factory. Some of these factories are metabolically more active than others. Fat cells are lazy and relatively inactive. They don't do much besides store energy; therefore, they don't burn much energy. Muscle cells, on the other hand, are dynamos of activity. They are constantly synthesizing new proteins, replicating DNA, contracting, and rebuilding. This constant stream of activity burns up a lot of calories.

Even at rest, muscle cells burn more calories than fat cells. This is a key concept in understanding your body's metabolism. No matter what you are doing, your muscle cells are more metabolically active than your fat cells, so they burn more calories.

Metabolism requires energy. Every cell in the body has a processing unit to tear down chemicals and another unit to assemble new compounds. There is a constant superhighway of traffic going on inside your cells. Chemicals are transported into the cell and end products are transported out. This constant transportation of materials requires energy.

Each and every cell conducts its business twenty-four hours a day, without time off or extra pay for overtime. They work all day, every day, whether you are at work or at rest.

The simple act of digesting food requires energy—a lot of energy. The body has to excrete enzymes, churn the intestines, break down all that food, and then move those food particles across the cell membranes of the intestine into the blood. Each of these activities requires energy.

This energy requirement is part of your basic metabolic rate, the energy needed daily to keep your heart pumping, your lungs breathing, your muscles contracting. This is energy you need to stay alive.

Excess energy is stored as fat. Food provides this energy to keep your body going. It also provides the building blocks for growth and replacement parts. The food that is not used for energy or as building blocks is converted by the body into storage forms for future use. A small amount is stored as *glycogen*, a natural starch. The rest is stored as fat.

The TriEnergetics Golden Rule of Metabolism

If you eat more calories than you metabolize, the excess will be stored in the body primarily as fat. If you burn more calories than you take in, you will mobilize your body's fat and you will lose weight.

This holds true no matter what kind of food you eat. Your food either gets utilized for energy or stored as fat. To understand why, let's look at what happens to food after it enters your mouth, when it is digested and processed by your body.

THE ART OF DIGESTION

Foods are made of water, fat, protein, carbohydrates, fiber, vitamins, and minerals. How do these compounds get into the body? We'll start with an overall view of digestion and follow a typical dinner from the time you place it in your mouth until its components end up in your cells.

Digestion begins with chewing and mixing the food with saliva. Saliva has an enzyme, *amylase,* that acts on starch to begin breaking it down. In this case, the amylase works on the bread, breaking down the carbohydrates to smaller molecules.

When you swallow, the bolus of food goes down the esophagus and into the stomach. There, everything you eat is churned and mixed together into a uniform broth. The steak is mixed with the potato, the corn, the bread, the pie, and the wine. When part of this mixture is sufficiently liquid, it is squirted into the small intestine. Any liquids you drink, particularly on an empty stomach, are apt to pass right through the stomach into the intestine, where they are absorbed. Solid foods may take hours to leave the stomach. Fats take the longest time of all.

The small intestine is the major food transportation station of the body. Here, the broth is mixed with bile from the liver, pancreatic enzymes, and enzymes formed in the wall of the intestine. The digested food, now in the form of tiny molecules, passes through the intestinal wall into the bloodstream. However, the intestine isn't a transparent membrane, and the food doesn't just diffuse through it. In order to get the food through this wall and into the bloodstream, your body must break the food down into small chemical units and actively transport them into the circulatory system. That transportation requires energy.

Once in the bloodstream, most of the food goes to the liver. The liver is the body's main food processing plant. It is also the main metabolic stabilizer of the body. It constantly monitors your blood sugar. When the blood sugar drops, the liver mobilizes some *glucose,* the natural sugar that is your body's basic fuel, and releases this sugar into the bloodstream.

Once the food has passed through the liver, the bloodstream carries the molecules through the capillaries, where those molecules are delivered to every cell in the body, absorbed, and utilized to fuel the cells' chemical furnaces.

Amazing, isn't it?

YOUR BODY'S NATURAL BIOCHEMISTRY

Now that we've traced the path of food from your mouth to the cells of your body, let's see how the body uses these nutrients. We're talking about your body's natural biochemistry.

Let's take a look at the major food groups and see where they fit into the metabolic scheme. By understanding how the food you eat is used, you'll see what type of foods will best feed the needs of your body.

CARBOHYDRATES

Let's start with the fun stuff: the carbs, sugars, starches. This is the stuff everyone loves to eat.

Carbohydrates are compounds of carbon, hydrogen, and oxygen. Every carbohydrate you eat, regardless of its complexity, is converted to glucose for use in the body. This means that whether you eat a potato, a pie, or whole-wheat bread, it all becomes glucose in the body.

Many people are under the impression that they need to avoid glucose in their diet. This is impossible. No matter what carbohydrate you eat, it will be made into glucose in the body. There's a reason for this. Glucose is the fuel that makes your body work. It's the gasoline in your engine.

Blood Sugar and Sugar Highs

Since all carbohydrates get converted to glucose during digestion, what difference is there between *simple sugars,* like candy, and *complex carbohydrates,* like whole grains? We're glad you asked.

The difference between eating a candy bar and eating a slice of whole-grain toast is in the speed with which the conversion to glucose is accomplished. Simple sugars, like candy, doughnuts, and cookies, take the glucose express highway into the bloodstream. Since they don't need to be broken down, they can pass rapidly through the stomach and are absorbed rapidly through the intestines. This causes a fast rise in your blood sugar, and this sugar surges through your bloodstream, giving you a "sugar high." This is why a breakfast of juice, sweetened coffee, and a doughnut gives you an immediate charge of energy in the morning.

But the energy doesn't last. Sensors in your body constantly monitor your blood sugar. When your blood sugar suddenly spikes, your pancreas secretes *insulin* to bring it down. The insulin forces the sugar out of the bloodstream and into the cells, where it can be used or stored. The problem is that when insulin is released in large amounts, there is usually an overcompensation in the sugar level, so the blood sugar plummets back down, sometimes dipping below the normal level. This dip is called the "sugar crash," or *hypoglycemia*.

The Sugar Trap

Hypoglycemia is a disturbance of the body's delicate balance, and it can have serious effects. Since the brain uses more glucose than any other organ, when the sugar drops, you feel tired, lethargic, sleepy, mentally drained, and listless. You feel more fatigued than if you'd never eaten the sugar-rich foods in the first place. Once the body senses that the sugar has fallen below a critical level, it tells the brain that there's a problem. The brain tries to solve the problem by telling you to eat something. This makes you feel hungry, and you grab some more food.

If you choose to eat another simple sugar, what happens? The same cycle is repeated. When you eat a diet high in simple sugars, you gain weight, feel tired, and continually overeat. Many people get caught in this sugar trap.

Seven Warning Signs of Hypoglycemia

▸ fatigue

▸ irritability

▸ hunger, even though you recently ate

▸ mental slowness

▸ forgetfulness

▸ inability to concentrate

▸ lethargy

The Insulin Weight Gain

By driving sugar from the bloodstream into the cells, insulin also predisposes you to gain weight. High insulin levels trigger the body to store the excess calories for later use, and that means fat. The higher your insulin levels, the more likely you are to store your excess calories as fat.

For Dynamic Energy, Eat Complex Carbohydrates

A good meal of complex carbohydrates, or carbohydrates eaten with other slowly digested foods like proteins, will keep your insulin levels normalized. Complex carbohydrates require more time to break down into small molecules, so you get a gradual and sustained absorption of glucose into your bloodstream. There is no sugar spike, so there is no massive release of insulin and no overcompensation hypoglycemia.

This slow infusion of nutrients will energize you, satisfy your hunger, and keep you going for hours. This is how you eat for dynamic energy. We recommend that you make complex carbohydrates the mainstay of your eating plan.

What Are Good Carbohydrate Foods?

When it comes to carbohydrates, select foods that are as unprocessed as possible. It is no coincidence that the national epidemic of obesity began at the same time as the appearance of processed snack, lunch, and dinner foods. Fifty years ago, there was no such thing as ready-to-eat microwave food, and the nation was much less fat. Now these foods and others like them are being touted as quick-and-easy meals. Don't buy into it.

Processing foods removes most of the micronutrients and fiber, leaving behind a high-calorie, nonnutritious husk. When whole grains are reduced to refined flour, they act like simple sugars. When you digest them, they crank up your insulin levels and launch you into the hypoglycemic sugar trap and weight gain.

Many people think that a glass of orange juice and a toasted bagel is a good breakfast. Not so. Yes, it is better than sweetened coffee and a doughnut, because there is less fat in a bagel than in a doughnut. But unless it's whole wheat, a bagel functions as a simple sugar, not a complex carbohydrate, and it gets converted to glucose rapidly. The result is that you get a sugar high, just as you would with sweet coffee and a doughnut.

Make it a point to select foods in their most natural state. Choose whole-grain breads and cereals. Try whole-grain pasta sprinkled with a low-fat, real cheese like parmesan rather than macaroni and cheese in a box. Natural or less processed foods retain more of their nutrients and will be less likely to wreak havoc on your insulin levels. You'll avoid the sugar trap and also gain less weight. The difference will be astonishing.

Not only that, but complex carbohydrates in the form of whole grains have a tremendous amount of B vitamins, which have an important role in preventing heart disease, and fiber, which reduces the risk of many cancers.

Good Carbohydrate Foods

There are many types of acceptable complex carbohydrates. Here's a list of the best choices for your daily meals.

- whole-grain breads
- vegetables
- corn
- oats
- lentils
- wild or brown rice
- peas
- sweet potatoes
- dried beans
- potatoes
- cereals (whole grain, not sugar coated)
- lima beans
- soybeans or tofu

These foods should be the backbone of your diet. Eat several servings of complex carbohydrates each day, supplemented with low-fat protein, like fish or chicken breast, and at least five to nine servings of vegetables and fruit.

Simple, processed carbohydrates should be avoided altogether—or, if you simply cannot give up these foods, eat them only once or twice per week.

When you buy a bread product, be careful. Many breads labeled "wheat bread" are made with refined wheat flour, not the whole grain. This is a simple carbohydrate. For the bread to be a healthy, complex-carbohydrate selection, it must say "whole grain." Look at the ingredient list. If it says "enriched wheat flour" or "wheat flour," it's probably not a whole-grain product. Look for "whole-wheat flour" instead.

Also, take care to select breads and crackers that have no more than two grams of fat per serving. Choose cereals with fewer than three grams of fat per serving. Be especially careful with granola-type cereals. They sound

Carbohydrate Foods to Eat Only in Moderation

> any product made from processed (refined) flour

> refined-flour breads, rolls, or buns

> processed crackers

> bagels made from white or processed flour

> simple-sugar foods like cookies, doughnuts, or candy

> pastries

> fried carbohydrates like french fries

> processed white-flour pasta

> sugary cereals

> any processed snack food

> ready-to-eat food

healthy, but many have more than 275 calories and seven grams of fat in a half-cup serving.

This leads us right to our next food group to discuss.

FATS

So, what are fats? Chemically, all fats are compounds comprising glycerol connected to one or more fatty acids. *Fatty acids* are an essential building block of your cell membranes and certain hormones. *Glycerol* is another name for glycerin. In structure it resembles glucose, and it behaves just like a carbohydrate in the body. Essentially, fats in the diet are just another source of glucose.

Fats require a lot of digestion before they can be mobilized as their basic molecules. For this reason, they stay in the stomach for a long time, making you feel full longer.

The American Diet: Too Much Fat

In the typical American diet, 40 to 60 percent of daily calories are derived from fat. If you eat the standard American diet (SAD), you are eating a diet far different from other societies, where people get over half their calories from vegetable products and fruits. We love our fat, and the reason is simple. Fatty foods taste good. The problem is, high-fat diets kill.

High-Fat Diets Cause Disease

We've all heard that high-fat diets cause heart disease. Then something like the high-protein, high-fat diet comes along, and suddenly everyone is gorging on fatty, greasy meats and claiming that it's healthy. What's the truth?

The truth is exactly what you thought. High-fat diets cause disease.

There is no disputing this point. People who eat less fat have a lower incidence of heart disease and cancers, including cancer of the breast and colon. This is one of the major flaws in the high-protein, high-fat, eat-what-you-want diets that have become so popular. By ingesting large amounts of animal protein and fat, people on these diets can easily top 60 percent of their daily caloric intake from fat. This can be deadly.

Even a good diet occasionally spiked with a high-fat meal is bad. In fact, a high-fat meal can have immediate adverse effects.

When you eat a high-fat meal, even if your diet is usually very healthy, you will get an immediate rise in your blood level of *factor VII*, a molecule that plays an important role in causing the blood to clot (Olsen et al. 2002). This increases the likelihood of a blood clot forming in your heart and causing a heart attack.

If you're healthy, you would probably have to eat about seventy to ninety grams of fat in one meal (that would be about two Big Macs) to get a significant increase in your blood level of factor VII. But if you have other risk factors for heart disease, even a small amount of fat can cause a significant rise.

A low-fat meal causes little or no immediate rise in factor VII.

Can You Eat Any Fat?

The National Institutes of Health have recommended that not more than 30 percent of the calories in your diet come from fat. Some coronary artery disease prevention programs, such as Dean Ornish's, restrict fat to no more than 10 percent of the total calories. Medically, this is a great idea, and Dr. Ornish has documented patients who have reversed coronary disease with his program of severe fat restriction. The problem is that it's really hard to stay on this diet. Most people try it for a while and then go back to their old habits.

The good news is that it's not necessary to cut all the fat out of your diet. In fact, you need to eat some fat. Fat is necessary to build your cell walls, and fat carries fat-soluble vitamins like D, E, A, and K. What you have to do is learn to eat the right amount of the right kinds of fats.

Some fats are good to eat any time, some are good only in small quantities, and others are never good to eat. In other words, there are a few good fats and a lot of bad fats.

Not All Fats Are Created Equal

The terms "saturated" and "unsaturated" fat are commonly used in food labeling. This classification is based on the number of hydrogen units in the fat. *Saturated fat* has no room for any more hydrogen to be attached. It is fully hydrogenated. *Unsaturated* fatty acids, on the other hand, have one or more locations where hydrogen blocks are missing. When only one pair of hydrogen blocks is missing, the fatty acid is *monounsaturated*. If there are two or more spots where a hydrogen pair is missing, the fat is *polyunsaturated*.

Bad fats: saturated fats. Saturated fats are bad because they clog your blood vessels, block off your blood supply, and cause heart attacks. Don't eat them if you can avoid them. If you don't know whether a fat is saturated, put it in the refrigerator. If it becomes hard and opaque, it is saturated. Animal products are the major source of saturated fat in the American diet, along with coconut and palm oils.

Seven Sources of Saturated Fats			
› fatty red meat	› cheese	› lard	› palm oil
	› butter	› coconut oil	› egg yolks

More bad fats: polyunsaturated fats. Polyunsaturated fats have been popular for a number of years because they are better for you than saturated fats. Unfortunately, there is a problem with polyunsaturated fats as well: they easily become rancid if heated or exposed to air for long periods, and rancid fats can cause cancer. A rancid fat is easy to detect. It smells bad, putrid. Do not eat any fatty food (such as nuts, chips, crackers, or cooking oil) that has a rancid odor. Don't reuse polyunsaturated fats that have been used for cooking, and don't buy polyunsaturated fats in containers too large to be used in a reasonable period of time.

There are a few good things about polyunsaturated fats. These fats are high in *linoleic* (omega-6) and *alpha-linolenic* (omega-3) oils. The body requires a small amount of these oils, and omega-3 may even help fight cancer and heart disease. But be careful. A little goes a long way. If your intake of omega-6 is high relative to omega-3, you can actually promote tumor growth.

We recommend that you eat polyunsaturated fats only in moderation. Use them sparingly in cooking.

Seven Sources of Polyunsaturated Fats	
‣ corn oil	‣ vegetable oil
‣ soybean oil	‣ flaxseed
‣ sesame oil	‣ cold-water fish
‣ safflower oil	

Even more bad fats: trans fats. *Trans fats* are the newest kid on the block. Technically, these aren't natural fats. They're what happens when you take vegetable oil and hydrogenate it, a process that makes stick margarine and solid shortening. This artificially created fat sends triglyceride and cholesterol levels through the roof, and it's a major culprit in clogging the arteries. If you see partially hydrogenated vegetable oil on the ingredient list, beware. We recommend that you avoid trans fats entirely. These are powerful artery cloggers.

Since trans fats are such a health hazard, the FDA issued a regulation in 2003 requiring all food manufacturers to list trans fats on the label. (The food manufacturers have until January 2006 to comply.) The FDA hopes that this will help people make healthier food choices and cut down their intake of trans fats. These trans fats are so deadly, the FDA estimates that in just three years after the labeling begins, 600 to 1,200 cases of coronary artery disease will be prevented and 250 to 500 deaths will be avoided.

Five Sources of Trans Fats

> packaged snacks

> stick margarine

> shortening

> peanut butter (not the natural kind, where the oil separates out)

> baked goods

Finally, a good fat: monounsaturated fat. Monounsaturated fats appear to be the safest fats to eat. In moderation, they do not increase the risk of cardiovascular disease, nor do they oxidize rapidly to become carcinogenic. They may even protect against cancer and heart disease. We recommend that you include an ample amount of these fats in your diet.

The best thing is that these fats are abundant in foods that are tasty and good for you. Monounsaturated fats can be found in legumes, vegetables, fish, and whole grains.

Seven Sources of Monounsaturated Fats

> olive oil

> canola oil

> olives

> peanuts

> avocados

> peas

> beans

> lentils

> fish

The Search for Hidden Fat

There is a lot of fat hidden in many foods, so you've got to read labels and look carefully at the fat content. Learn to search out the hidden fat. The labels can be misleading. Many items (including dressings, sauces, cookies, potato chips, and popcorn) are labeled as lean, light, and low fat when they are not.

Let us show you what we mean. A name-brand gourmet popcorn is advertised as containing one-third less calories, fat, and oil. Sounds great! Let's look at the label.

NUTRITION INFORMATION (PER SERVING)	
Serving size	9.5 g
Servings per bag	18
Calories	35
Protein	1 g
Carbohydrate	6 g
Fat	2 g

Still look good? Two grams of fat certainly looks small, doesn't it? But if you calculate the amount of calories that are coming from this "small" amount of fat, you find a completely different story.

It's a fact that each gram of fat has nine calories, so let's calculate two grams of fat times nine calories per gram. That equals eighteen calories. So eighteen calories per serving come from fat. Doesn't sound too bad. But a serving only has thirty-five calories. That means if you divide eighteen by thirty-five, you get 51 percent. That means that 51 percent of the calories in this popcorn comes from fat.

Is that low fat? We don't think so. This popcorn may have one-third less fat than the regular variety, but it is still half fat. Imagine the amount of fat in the regular popcorn.

This brings up a very important point about fat. Fat not only contains over twice the calories of protein or carbohydrate but also contains very little water. This means that there are about as many calories in one gram of fat as there are in five grams of lean meat.

How to Search for Hidden Fat

Here's how to calculate the percentage of calories in a food that comes from fat. Read the label carefully, then

1. Multiply the number of fat grams per serving by nine calories per gram. This gives you the fat calories in the food.

2. Divide this number by the total number of calories per serving. This will give you the percentage of calories in each serving that comes from fat.

Why Do Humans Have Body Fat?

You know that bears store fat because they hibernate all winter and live off their fat, but what about you?

Humans also store fat, and perhaps you know from personal experience that you do it easily. Your body makes fat from protein and carbohydrate and stores it in the most visible places. Does this corpulence have a purpose, or is it a punishment for eating too much?

The answer is that fat serves a purpose. It is a reservoir of energy for your body to use in an emergency. In this regard, you are like a bear. Unfortunately, your metabolism is a little different than a bear's. When a bear hibernates and doesn't eat, it burns mostly fat for fuel. When you diet and try to lose weight by not eating, your body burns mostly muscle. The fat is the last to go. This may not be fair, but it is the way your body works.

However, it's possible to train your body to burn more fat by exercising. During aerobic exercise, the muscles of a well-conditioned person derive 70 percent of the energy they need from fat, while 30 percent comes from sugar. A person who is not well conditioned primarily burns sugar and very little fat. The more you exercise, the more fat you burn.

Our Fat Recommendations

Here are our basic recommendations about fat.

The bulk of your calories should come from complex carbohydrates, not fat. Eat lots of fruits, whole grains, legumes, vegetables, and nonfat dairy products. Eat small servings of low-fat, high-protein foods, like skinless chicken or turkey breast. Eat cheeses in moderation. Always choose fat-free dairy.

The majority of your fat intake should be monounsaturated fats. Replace butter with a high-monounsaturated oil like canola or olive oil. Avoid the saturated fats like the plague.

Eat fish once or twice a week. The omega-3 fatty acids in fish oils are protective against heart disease.

Eliminate or cut back hydrogenated oils. Avoid packaged foods, stick margarine, crackers, cookies, puddings, and potato chips. Remember, hydrogenation creates trans fats, which can greatly boost your cholesterol and cause heart disease.

The TriEnergetics Fat Guide		
Good Oils	**Great Fish Sources of Good Omega-3 Oils**	**Butter or Margarine?**
› canola		
› flaxseed		› Avoid stick margarine.
› olive	› salmon	
› walnut	› mackerel	› Avoid butter.
Bad Oils	› tuna	› Choose tub margarine or Benecol, a butter substitute.
› coconut	› trout	
› corn	› sardines	
› safflower	› herring	
› palm		

PROTEINS

Proteins are all the rage right now, as many people are flocking to the high-protein, low-carbohydrate diet, so let's take a close look at proteins and see how they're used in the body and how much of them you really need.

Many people think that they will become stronger and build more muscle by eating a lot of protein. Americans like the idea of getting muscular without exerting themselves too much. Unfortunately, it doesn't work that way. Muscle does not grow like a weed. You can't fertilize it with protein and watch it grow. You must exercise a muscle if you want it to grow.

What Are Proteins?

Proteins are long chains of amino acids connected together. *Amino acids* are similar to glucose but contain nitrogen molecules, which are essential for building and repairing cells and tissues.

Amino acids can be used either for energy or as building blocks for tissue. When the body is starved, the liver's supply of glycogen rapidly gets depleted, and the body will break down fats and muscle for energy. So protein and amino acids can be converted to glucose and used in the body.

One advantage of eating a lot of protein is that the protein takes longer to digest than complex carbohydrates. This means that protein provides an even slower sustained release of energy. Also, since protein takes longer to digest, it stays in the stomach longer and you'll feel full longer.

How Much Protein Do You Need?

Most Americans eat much more protein than they need. You should take in enough protein to satisfy your body's needs, but if you eat more protein than you need, the excess is converted to your nemesis, fat.

How much protein does the average adult need? Twenty-five to thirty grams a day is adequate.

Let's relate this figure to your daily life. A glass of milk has eight grams of protein, an egg has six grams, and a slice of whole-wheat toast has two grams, so a hearty breakfast can supply almost all of your daily protein needs. A small serving of steak, about the size of a McDonald's hamburger, has twenty-five grams of protein. If you have a big breakfast, an adequate lunch, and a normal dinner, you are probably way over your basic daily protein needs.

If you exercise vigorously and are attempting to build muscle, your protein needs will increase to seventy to eighty grams a day. That's all.

> ### Daily Protein Needs
>
> The average adult needs only about twenty-five grams of protein a day.
>
> An adult who exercises vigorously needs up to eighty grams of protein a day.

Get Fat the High-Protein Way

Eating extra protein won't give you a protein reserve for building more muscle. Remember, a calorie is a calorie whether it comes from protein or carbohydrates. If you eat more protein than your body needs, the excess will be converted to fat.

What's more, too much protein may be dangerous to your health. When you eat protein, its digestion makes by-products that are converted to urea and excreted by your kidneys. If you take in too much protein, you put a tremendous strain on the kidneys that can cause kidney stones or even kidney disease.

The high-protein diet being touted these days is also high in fat, which makes it a particularly bad diet. While you might lose weight initially on this diet, the combination of high protein and high fat can be devastating for your health.

Should Humans Eat Animal Protein?

In addition to their love of fatty foods, many Americans are addicted to meat. The mere thought of meatless living is too much for many to bear.

Perhaps this is why the high-protein diet became so popular—it allowed many people to eat what they loved and still think that they were healthy.

Unfortunately, that's not the case.

The honest truth is that human beings were never designed to be primarily meat eaters. One simple way to prove this fact is to look at the human digestive system and see what it was designed to handle. Meat eaters, like tigers or lions, have sharp teeth for tearing and shredding and short intestines to rapidly excrete the waste that comes with eating meat.

We don't. Humans—like most plant eaters—have molars, designed primarily for grinding and chewing, and an intestinal system that is more than forty feet long to allow us to absorb as many nutrients as possible from our vegetarian food. Our entire anatomical and physiological makeup shows that we were primarily designed to eat plants.

But don't take our word for it. Look at any human society that hasn't been inundated by Westernized culture and you'll see that their diets are primarily plant based, occasionally sprinkled with meat.

Why are we different? Somewhere along the way, humans in Western society decided that they loved the taste of meat. Further, they decided that meat could be eaten at any meal, several times a day, in combination with any other foods. There is no other animal in the world that eats this way. But we do.

The Skinny on Meat

In the TriEnergetics program, we don't advocate that you give up eating meat. If you choose to eat only a vegan diet, that's your decision. But if not, don't worry. There can be a role for animal protein in your diet; you just have to know exactly what you're getting yourself into.

Eating meat has been clearly associated with an increased risk of cancer. People who eat red meat five or more times a week have four times the risk of getting colon cancer than people who eat meat only once a month (Chao, Thun, and Connell 2005). Animal meats, as a general rule, are high in saturated fats. Also, since our digestive tracts weren't primarily designed for meat, eating too much animal protein can cause a whole host of digestive problems.

Beware Hidden Fat in Meat

Ground beef is the third biggest source of saturated fat in the average American diet, behind cheese and whole milk. The problem with ground beef is that the labels can be very misleading, allowing you to eat a tremendous amount of fat even when you think you are making healthy choices.

Let's take a look at this. If you go to the market and select a lean cut of ground beef, the label may say "80 percent lean." Sounds good, but it's not. What this really means is that the beef is 80 percent lean by weight, not by caloric content. Twenty percent of the beef, by weight, is fat. In terms of calories, this means that the "80 percent lean" ground beef actually contributes 70 percent of its calories in fat.

Here's a table to help you determine how many calories from fat you are getting when you buy ground beef. This table reflects the caloric content of a three-and-a-half-ounce raw beef patty.

CALORIES FROM FAT IN LEAN GROUND BEEF	
Percent of Fat by Weight	Percent of Calories from Fat
10% (90% lean beef)	51%
15% (85% lean beef)	61%
20% (80% lean beef)	70%
25% (75% lean beef)	75%

So, What Protein Should You Eat?

In the TriEnergetics program, we will gently guide you toward a less meat-intensive diet. When you do eat meat, we recommend that you eat primarily poultry, fish, and lean red meats.

Don't worry that you won't get enough protein in your diet if you decrease your meat consumption. There's more than enough protein in grains, beans, and legumes to satisfy your daily needs. It doesn't matter to your body whether the protein you take in was originally steak, chicken, fish, or soybeans. An amino acid from one is indistinguishable from another. It's all the same after it's metabolized and broken down by the body.

Moving On

Now that you have a better understanding of how your body metabolizes food, you're ready to eat in a way that generates dynamic energy and improves your health. Let's go on to the next chapter and see how you can do this.

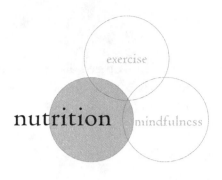

exercise

nutrition mindfulness

chapter 5

The TriEnergetics Approach:
Eating for Dynamic Energy

The power of eating well cannot be overemphasized. How you eat has a greater impact on your body than anything else you can do. Even more important than exercise is the fuel, the nutrients, and the vitamins that you take in.

The problem with eating is that people are confused. Americans are bombarded with so much information every day that the message gets lost in the words. Add to that the fact that the food industry and the diet industry have been dishing out misinformation for years, insisting that their product or diet plan is healthy, and it's no wonder people are confused.

But let's not throw out the baby with the bathwater. Scientists have learned a tremendous amount about how the body functions and what foods and what nutrients the body needs to maintain optimal health and wellness. Research has revealed what nutrients can strengthen the immune system, cleanse the arteries, purify toxins, build strong bones, and calm the nerves.

We've created the TriEnergetics nutritional plan to sift through the half-truths and give you an easy-to-understand, simple-to-follow plan for eating for optimal health. This plan is based on the best nutritional science and has been tested and proven to be effective in our seminars.

This is the truth about how to feed your body for dynamic energy.

EATING MADE EASY

In the TriEnergetics program, we don't insist that you follow a specific diet. You don't need to weigh food or calculate fat content. Instead, we suggest that you make a lifestyle change. To help you reach this goal, each week we'll suggest one simple adjustment in your eating habits. The cumulative effect of these small changes—along with the exercise routines and meditation practices—will be a dramatic improvement in your health and appearance. The effectiveness of this holistic, incremental approach has been proven time and time again.

Within a few weeks of starting our program, the majority of participants notice incredible improvements in their energy level and their health, as well as a reduction in body fat, strengthened muscles, and less stress.

● Mary's Turnaround

Mary had tried every diet under the sun. She'd been on the grapefruit diet, the cabbage soup diet, the sugar-busters diet, and the 1,200-calorie diet. With each of these radical diet changes, she lost weight—sometimes an impressive amount of weight—but invariably the weight came right back on. She tried fen-phen, but stopped when she learned that the drugs could cause serious health problems. Most recently, she'd been on the Atkins diet, and while she lost weight on it, she felt run-down and listless. Within two weeks of stopping the Atkins diet, she regained all of the twenty pounds she'd lost.

Near her wits' end, Mary enrolled in the TriEnergetics program. We taught her how to eat naturally, using her body's metabolism to bolster her dynamic energy. She also learned the importance of balancing all three of her natural energies—her nourishment, mind, and body.

By the end of the six-week program, Mary had lost fifteen pounds, not from dieting but from modifying her lifestyle. She now exercised regularly and meditated daily, and she had never felt better in her life. Her energy had skyrocketed, and her stress level had plummeted.

EATING THEN AND NOW

Our ancestors, like all living creatures, ate to survive. Eating was a simple, fundamental behavior. If there was enough food, people stored the excess for a time when it would be needed. What foods they ate depended upon what they could grow, scavenge, or hunt. Their diets were primarily grains and fruits, supplemented with whatever meat could be obtained. The food was organic and unprocessed.

Today, food is readily available, but it is highly processed, high in fat, high in calories, high in sugar, and full of additives. Highly advanced technologies make it easy to produce too many foods with too little nutritional value. The American way of eating has made it too easy to get fat and become unhealthy. Stress, time pressures, and fast foods all share responsibility.

Given how hard they had to work for their limited food supply, our ancestors couldn't afford to eat to feed their emotions. But the abundance of food in modern America—and way it's marketed—encourages us to use food to satisfy our emotional as well as physical needs.

INTEGRATING YOUR MIND AND YOUR EATING

In order to control your weight and eat for optimum health, it is important that you learn to integrate your mind and your eating. In our supercharged society, people are hardly aware of *what* they're eating, much less *why* they're eating. Modern humans still eat because we are hungry, but we also eat for many other reasons.

What about you?

Think about the reasons you eat. Do you eat when you are bored, when you are unhappy, when you are frustrated, when you go to the movies, when you are out with friends? Perhaps this sounds familiar: someone brings a box of cookies or doughnuts to work, and instinctively you reach for one, only to regret it later.

How often do you eat in front of the television or while talking with your partner? How often do you overeat because you haven't been paying attention to what's going into your mouth? How often have you finished a meal and felt stuffed, even uncomfortable?

Eating unconsciously has become a major problem in our fast-paced society. A quarter of all meals are eaten in the car. That's no way to live. How many of your meals are gobbled down at your desk at work or forced into tiny time slots between other parts of your busy day?

One of the most powerful changes you can make is to pay attention to your eating. You can learn to stop eating once your hunger has been satisfied. Pay attention to your body. It will tell you when you've had enough to eat.

Let's take a look at how to integrate your mind and your eating.

UNDERSTAND WHY YOU EAT

Many people overeat because they are bored, tired, or depressed. These mental states can have a tremendous impact on your eating. Take the time to recognize which, if any, of these emotions are influencing your habits and causing you to eat unconsciously. Later in this section, we'll teach you two techniques to help you take back control of your eating.

MANAGE YOUR STRESS

Stress increases your body's production of *cortisol,* a very powerful hormone that can redirect your fat stores. The more stressed you are, the more likely you are to store fat in your middle. In order to control this, you must learn how to beat stress. The TriEnergetics stress management techniques will have a profound effect on your ability to control your eating and your weight.

MAINTAIN A POSITIVE SELF-IMAGE

It does you no good to criticize and condemn yourself for being overweight. All this will do is sap you of your natural dynamic energy, leaving you feeling lethargic and depressed. Quiet the critic that lives inside of you. Maintain a positive self-image by taking steps toward controlling your weight problem with the TriEnergetics approach to exercise, nutrition, and stress management.

SHED A NEW LIGHT ON YOUR FOOD

Stop thinking about food as being either good or bad. Instead, think about food as fuel for your body. Rather than agonizing over dieting, focus on nourishing your body. This will help you make better food choices. The Eating for Nourishment exercise will help you along this path.

How to Integrate Your Mind and Your Eating

› Understand why you eat.

› Manage your stress.

› Maintain a positive self-image.

› Shed a new light on your food.

EXERCISE: Eating for Nourishment

The goal of this exercise is quite simple: to make you aware of everything that you put in your mouth. This is a great way to stop yourself from eating that doughnut before you regret it.

Each time you reach for a food, whether during a meal or as a snack, ask yourself one simple question: *Will this food nourish me?* If the answer is yes, go for it. If not, don't.

You'll be surprised at how powerful this exercise can be. Just by taking that extra moment and focusing your attention on your food, you empower yourself to take charge of your eating and make better choices. More often than not, asking that simple question will prevent you from eating something that you would regret later. Your body instinctively knows what's healthy and what isn't.

Another wonderful exercise that we'd like to share with you is mindful eating. This exercise is designed to help you savor your food and not overeat. It also serves as a great meditative technique.

The concept of mindfulness is based upon ancient Taoist teachings. Being mindful simply means being aware. Mindful eating means concentrating on everything you are eating for every moment you are eating.

It may be a challenge to you to eat this way, because it's different from the way that you have always eaten. Look upon mindful eating as an exercise that you will practice to heighten your awareness of your eating habits.

To eat mindfully, you need to concentrate on every bite of food that enters your mouth. This means that you can't be doing something else while you're eating. Turn off the TV. Don't read the newspaper or cereal box. Don't talk with your partner, children, friends, or coworkers.

It will be tough at first. If you're like most people, you've been talking, reading, or watching television at almost every meal since you were a child. This lack of attention to what's been going into your mouth may be one of the reasons you have trouble keeping your weight in control.

Only practice mindful eating when you can be alone, when you feel focused, and when you have the time. If you try to rush through the meal, it won't work.

EXERCISE: Mindful Eating

Before you start eating, sit quietly and close your eyes for a few minutes, allowing yourself to relax. Take a deep, calming breath. Now open your eyes and focus on the food in front of you. Continue to breathe slowly and deeply while you take a small portion from your plate. Chew slowly, savoring the subtle sensations of the food as it touches your taste buds.

If you're eating an orange, take a small bite from one of the sections and let the tart citrus taste linger in your mouth. Note the texture of the orange, the coolness of the fruit, and the tingling sensation in your mouth. Eat very slowly, concentrating on every bite. Do the same with the other foods that you are eating.

Pay attention to how your stomach feels. It will signal to you when your hunger has been satisfied. You'll be amazed to realize how much food you normally eat between the time your hunger has been satisfied and the time your stomach is full. When you eat mindfully, you learn to stop eating when you are no longer hungry.

This exercise is simple, and it is powerful. After just a few sessions, you'll be keenly aware of how much you're eating and what you're eating. When you concentrate your awareness on your food, you'll find that you gravitate naturally toward healthier selections because they make you feel better. You'll also find that you don't need to eat nearly as much food to be satisfied.

As simple as this exercise sounds, it isn't easy to do in the real world. Distractions and time pressure make it difficult to take the time to concentrate on something as simple as eating. But try it. Play with it a few times; practice it until you learn to be in tune with your body. We believe you'll find it infinitely rewarding.

EATING THE TRIENERGETICS WAY

We want you to look better, feel better, be healthier, and have more energy. We say that eating should be a complete experience. Forget about weighing and measuring your food. Forget about diets; diets don't work. We want to give you an integrated eating plan that will maximize the nourishment of your body.

You need to eat. Enjoy eating. Eat with gusto and eat for your pleasure. Of greatest importance, eat to generate dynamic energy.

EATING MADE EASY

As you learned in the last chapter, the foundation of the TriEnergetics nourishment plan is a diet high in complex carbohydrates for sustained energy, low in processed sugars to avoid the sugar highs and lows, moderate in protein for sustenance, and low in fat to reduce your risk of heart disease and cancer.

Here's how it looks, meal by meal.

BREAKFAST

Eat breakfast every morning to provide energy to start the day. Breakfast should be high in complex carbohydrates (like whole grains) and low in simple sugars (like doughnuts). This will provide a steady blood sugar level all morning and prevent the late-morning blahs. The addition of some protein (such as smoked salmon, low-fat cottage cheese, or egg substitutes) will help stave off late-morning hunger.

SNACKING

If you do get hungry, snack on complex-carbohydrate, low-sugar foods. Avoid quick fixes like doughnuts, pastries, or bagels. Try dried fruits, fresh fruits, yogurt, whole-grain breads, soybeans, or raw, unsalted peanuts or almonds.

LUNCH

Lunch is a good time to eat some protein in addition to your complex carbs. Some of the amino acids will promote alertness and satisfy your hunger. Salad or vegetables will provide good carbohydrates and some protein.

DINNER

We recommend a moderate, healthy dinner. On the TriEnergetics plan, we will move you slowly away from meat-based dinners to more vegetable-based dinners, including pastas, soups, salads, and casseroles. It's generally not a good idea to eat much just before bedtime. Rather, eat a light dinner, then allow time for your body to digest your food before sleep.

DESSERT

One of the surest ways to remove unnecessary calories from your diet is to eliminate desserts. However, if you absolutely crave it, by all means eat a little dessert. It's always better to eat a little of something than to deprive yourself until the craving becomes so strong that you binge.

When you do eat dessert, try to keep it in moderation. Share with others; skip the sauces, syrups, and whipped cream that often accompany dessert; and try to save the really rich desserts for special occasions. Sherbets are a better choice than ice cream or frozen yogurt. Fresh berries or fruit make a truly healthy dessert.

DRINKING

Many people like to finish off their day with an alcoholic drink or two. Can you do this while maintaining a healthy lifestyle? The answer is yes and no.

Research indicates that an occasional glass or two of wine (preferably red) may indeed be beneficial (Tsang et al. 2005). Wine is naturally chock-full of antioxidants that may reduce your risk of heart disease and cancer.

But this doesn't mean you should start drinking like a fish. Alcohol is surprisingly high in calories. A small shot of vodka has about 60 calories, and a full bottle of beer can have 200 calories or more. Microbrewery beers are even more fattening. Many people will hesitate at eating a piece of cheesecake but think nothing of throwing back two or three drinks after work. Too much alcohol can also rob the body of vitamins and minerals. So while an occasional glass or two of wine may be healthy, alcohol should not be a regular part of your lifestyle.

> ### The TriEnergetics Guide to Eating for Health and Vitality
>
> **Breakfast.** Choose complex carbohydrates, plus some protein (such as eggs, egg substitute, or smoked salmon).
>
> **Snacking.** Choose complex-carbohydrate, low-sugar foods, like dried fruits, fresh fruits, yogurt, or whole-grain breads.
>
> **Lunch.** Choose protein in addition to complex carbs.
>
> **Dinner.** Choose moderate, vegetarian, or light-meat dinners including pastas, soups, salads, and casseroles.
>
> **Dessert.** Eat desserts in moderation, or select fresh berries or fruit.
>
> **Drinking.** Drink alcohol only in moderation (one or two glasses of wine per week).

EAT YOUR VEGGIES

Vegetables are a wonderful source of nutrients, fiber, and complex carbohydrates. In the course of the six-week TriEnergetics program, you'll be adding more vegetables to your diet. Here are two important things to consider.

EATING VEGETABLES RAW IS NOT ALWAYS BEST

Exposure to heat can denature some of the vitamins, but briefly heating high-fiber vegetables such as broccoli can release powerful phytochemicals.

FRESH VEGETABLES ARE NOT ALWAYS HEALTHIEST

Produce can lose much of its disease-fighting power during the first two weeks after being picked, while it sits at the warehouse, at your supermarket, and in your refrigerator. So unless you know that your produce is locally grown and freshly picked, you're better off with frozen vegetables, which are preserved right after harvesting.

Now here's the A-list of veggies.

Broccoli. Loaded with antioxidants, this vegetable is the big winner. Broccoli has good supplies of vitamin C, folic acid, calcium, fiber, alpha-lipoic acid, genistein, sulforaphane, isothiocyanates, coenzyme Q_{10}, lutein, and carotenoids. It is best prepared in the microwave or steamed to coax out the cancer-fighting phytochemicals.

Carrots. Carrots are high in vitamin C, calcium, fiber, and carotenoids. Microwave or steam them to free the phytochemicals.

Cabbage. Cabbage is high in vitamin C, indoles, isothiocyanates, and carotenoids. Eat it raw in salads. Shred it just before serving to minimize exposure to light and air, which inactivates the vitamins.

Greens (mustard, collard, or turnip greens; kale; chard). Greens are high in vitamin C, flavonoids, and B vitamins. Microwave or steam these for best flavor.

Beans and legumes (soybeans, kidney beans, chickpeas, lentils). Beans and legumes are high in folic acid, isoflavones, genistein, B vitamins, and vitamin E. Cook these and add them to soups, casseroles, stews, and salads.

Tomatoes. Tomatoes are high in vitamin C, carotenoids, and lycopene. Eat them raw, drink them puréed as a juice, or simmer them in homemade sauces.

Spinach. Popeye was right about this one. Spinach is packed with folate, beta carotene, magnesium, lutein, and fiber. Eat it raw in salads or cooked in lasagna or casseroles.

AN APPLE A DAY

A good selection of fruits is essential for a healthy diet. When looking at which fruits to eat, the best choices are

- prunes

- raisins

- blueberries

- strawberries

- apples

- red grapes

- plums

To learn more about these wonderful, disease-fighting foods, read Steven Pratt's book, *Superfoods: Fourteen Foods That Will Change Your Life* (William Morrow, 2004). In this excellent resource, Pratt discusses in detail those foods that pack the most nutritional punch per bite.

TRIENERGETICS AND THE NEW FOOD PYRAMID

The TriEnergetics program has been carefully designed to help you feel better and stay healthier. We are very pleased to see that the new food guidelines developed by the U.S. Department of Agriculture and supported by the Department of Health and Human Services agree with our recommendations. The seven USDA guidelines for a healthful diet are

- Eat a variety of foods.

- Balance the food you eat with physical activity.

- Choose a diet with plenty of grain products, vegetables, and fruits.

- Choose a diet low in fat, saturated fat, and cholesterol.

- Choose a diet moderate in sugars.

- Choose a diet moderate in salt.

- If you drink alcoholic beverages, do so in moderation.

THE TRUTH ABOUT FIBER

Much has been written—and much controversy has been created— about fiber. Here's the real story.

Fiber protects the heart. High-fiber foods lower bad (LDL) cholesterol, blood pressure, and *triglycerides* (potentially harmful lipids in the blood). This protects against heart disease. A study by Liu and colleagues (2002) showed that women who ate twenty-three grams of fiber a day were 23 percent less likely to have a heart attack than women who ate only eleven grams a day. The results were even more impressive in men, who reduced their risk of heart attack by 36 percent on the high-fiber diet.

Fiber fights cancer. Almost every study looking for a link between fiber and cancer has shown that a high-fiber diet is protective against cancer. This is especially true for colon cancer, the second most common cancer in America. High-fiber diets have been shown to be protective against breast, rectal, stomach, thyroid, and mouth cancers as well.

In the past, there has been some confusion over the role of fiber in preventing colon cancer, but two studies recently published in the *Lancet* offer new insight.

In the first study (Peters et al. 2003), researchers at the National Cancer Institute looked at the diet of 34,000 participants. All were free of precancerous colorectal polyps when the trial began. The researchers found that those participants eating a high-fiber diet (thirty-six grams or more of fiber each day) were 25 percent less likely to develop polyps than those eating fewer than twelve grams.

The other study (Bingham et al. 2003) looked at 520,000 people in ten European countries. This study found a 25 percent reduced rate in colorectal cancer in those participants eating about thirty-five grams of fiber daily compared with those eating less than fifteen grams. The study also showed that the low-fiber eaters could reduce their risk of colon cancer by 40 percent simply by doubling their intake of fiber—another bit of really good news.

Fiber helps you lose weight. Adults on a high-fiber diet gain less weight than those on a low-fiber diet. This is because fiber suppresses insulin, and lower insulin means less hunger and less eating.

Fiber aids digestion. There's no disputing this one. A high-fiber diet promotes digestion and reduces constipation and diarrhea. A high-fiber diet is also essential for preventing *diverticulosis* (the formation of abnormal pouches in the intestinal wall). Furthermore, a high-fiber diet reduces the risk of ulcers and gallstones.

Fiber helps keep you alive and healthy. Woodward, Tunstall-Pedoe, and Bolton-Smith (1999) found that women who ate a high-fiber diet reduced their risk of premature death from all causes by 33 percent compared to women who ate diets low in fiber. That makes fiber an even more powerful reducer of mortality than antioxidants.

The Truth About Fiber

> Fiber protects the heart.

> Fiber fights cancer.

> Fiber helps you lose weight.

> Fiber aids digestion.

> Fiber helps keep you alive and healthy.

TRIENERGETICS AND FIBER

The TriEnergetics eating plan is designed to help you gradually increase the amount of natural soluble and insoluble fiber in your diet. Both soluble and insoluble fiber go undigested when you eat them; therefore, they're not absorbed into the bloodstream. Instead of being used for energy, fiber is excreted from your body.

Soluble fiber prolongs stomach emptying time, so sugar is released and absorbed more slowly, and it lowers total and LDL cholesterol. It can be found in oats, oat bran, legumes, fruits, whole grains, and flaxseed.

Insoluble fiber promotes regular bowel movements, keeps the pH level in the intestines healthy, and removes toxic waste through the colon. Insoluble fiber comes mainly from wheat bran, whole-wheat products, corn bran, flaxseed, green beans, cauliflower, potato skins, and the skins of fruits and root vegetables.

Many of the fad diets, like the high-protein diet, sacrifice fiber by outlawing whole grains and concentrating on fatty, low-fiber animal proteins. This can be deadly.

On the TriEnergetics program, you'll slowly increase the amount of vegetables and whole grains that you eat, while reducing the junk and fatty meats that are low in fiber. This is a natural, healthy way to eat.

AND FINALLY, EAT LESS

As a whole, our society eats too much. Portions are too big, and most people eat too often. No other society consumes as much food as in the United States, and no other society suffers from the same high rate of obesity. In addition, many people have become too dependent on food as a nurturing diversion from stress. And they may not be conscious of all the food that they place in their mouths.

All of this adds up to a fat country.

It is important that you take back control of your eating. Several studies have shown a direct correlation between eating less and having a longer, healthier life. You may find it difficult to reduce your food intake, but there are some easy skills you can learn to trim down the amount that you eat without feeling deprived or hungry. We're not talking about dieting. We've already shown you that dieting doesn't work. We are simply talking about not overeating.

We all do it—eat too much, then hold our stomachs and moan that we ate too much—but most overeating isn't this dramatic. Most overeating is simply finishing that one extra piece of pie or eating that last bite on the plate or reaching into the box for one more cookie.

Most of the time, people do these things not because they're hungry, but because it is a habit. Unfortunately, this habit can pack on the pounds.

Here are eight tips to help you reduce the amount of food that you eat.

Eat several small meals throughout the day rather than one or two large meals. This will help maintain a steady blood sugar level and prevent extreme hunger when your sugars are too low.

Never eat right out of the box, bag, or carton. Always serve yourself a portion and put the box away.

Don't eat meals family style. Rather than serving the food on platters on the table, leave the food on the stove. Place a serving on your plate and sit down at the table.

Practice mindful eating. Learn to become aware of when your body's hunger is satisfied. You'll appreciate your food more and be less inclined to overeat.

Snack heartily on fruits and vegetables. Eat as much of these foods as you like. These low-calorie foods will fill you up and prevent you from overeating other foods.

Don't eat in front of the TV or computer. When you eat, make it a separate activity so you can concentrate better on the amounts you eat.

Don't finish everything on your plate. Often, your eyes are bigger than your stomach, and you have to force that last bit of food into your mouth. You don't need to do this. Always leave a little bit of food on your plate.

Remind yourself to eat less. This will make you more aware of the amount that you are eating.

EAT FOR HEALTH

So far, we've discussed how you must balance the energy derived from foods with your body's physical energy needs, and how you must learn to quiet your mind in order to control your unconscious eating habits.

The TriEnergetics program will help you focus on eating for dynamic energy. When you do, you will find that

- You don't need to count calories.

- You can eat almost any amount of the recommended foods.

- You will have more sustained energy.

- You will lose weight.

- You will feel better.

When you start the program, you'll find that each week we'll offer a suggestion for modifying one of your unhealthy eating habits. Each suggestion is easy to follow and concise.

Stay with the program, and within a few weeks you'll notice a wonderful change in the way you look and in the way you feel.

Enjoy the change.

TEN TRIENERGETICS GOLDEN RULES FOR EATING FOR DYNAMIC ENERGY AND BETTER HEALTH

1. Enjoy eating. It's a pleasure, not a punishment.

   In order to develop permanent good habits, you must make permanent changes. It's essential that you like what you are doing. This is not a diet but a way of life. You will succeed because you have set a goal of feeling better and improving your health. You will need to give up some of the foods that you've been eating, but there are many others from which to choose.

2. Eat less.

   We've just discussed several ways that you can avoid overeating. One is to eat several smaller meals throughout the day, rather than one or two large meals. Try to take your largest meal at lunch, and always eat something for breakfast.

   Never eat right out of the package. It's hard to monitor how much you ingest that way. Don't eat your meals family style, with the serving platters on the table. Rather, dish out your portion and carry your plate to the table.

Finally, don't forget to practice mindful eating. This will help you get in touch with your body's true need for food and help you to stop overeating.

3. **Do not add oils or fats to your food.**
Avoid eating margarine, mayonnaise, butter, oily salad dressings, and cream cheese. We want you to keep your fat calories down to 30 percent or less of your daily caloric intake. This is no small order, since the typical American diet is 40 to 50 percent fat. You don't need to count calories or weigh foods. If you follow our simple suggestions, you will meet this goal. When you do add oil, stick to the monounsaturated oils.

4. **Eat all of the fruit and vegetables you want.**
You can't go wrong with these guys. Dark green vegetables are good for your heart. Red and orange veggies are good also. Fruits are a great source of fiber and vitamins. The USDA recommends nine servings of fruit or vegetables a day. Most Americans don't come near this goal.

Remember to watch out for the creamy, fatty dressings on your salads. Try any of the oil-free salad dressings, or use a little olive oil and vinegar on your fresh salads.

Some vegetables actually require more calories to digest than are contained in the food. You can lose weight by eating alfalfa sprouts, broccoli, cabbage, celery, cucumber, lettuce, mushrooms, and radishes.

5. **Become more of a vegetarian.**
If a completely vegetarian diet isn't your cup of tea, make a few compromises. Eat more poultry and fish. Stop looking for the beef, but when you must have that piece of meat, eat a lean cut.

6. **Snack with discretion.**
What do we mean? Most snack foods are dangerous to your health as well as your waistline. We suggest snacking on

fruits and vegetables. Try dried apricots instead of chocolate and celery sticks instead of potato chips. What a difference this will make! Try baby carrots, fresh fruits, or dried fruits.

At times you may crave carbohydrate snacks. When this urge hits you, avoid the doughnut boxes and cookie bags and instead opt for whole-grain breads, pretzels, or air-popped popcorn.

7. **Fat free does not mean healthy.**
"Fat free" on the label does not mean calorie free or even low calorie. Many fat-free foods make up for the lack of fat with a ton of extra sugar. High sugar content equals high calorie content. We've known many people who have packed on the weight by eating "fat-free" snacks.

You can always calculate what percentage of a food's calories come from fat by multiplying the number of fat grams by nine, then dividing this number by the total calories per serving. You'll be amazed how fatty "low-fat" foods are.

8. **Eat complex carbohydrates whenever you can.**
Complex carbohydrates are good for your metabolism and good for you. Eat plenty of legumes, beans, and whole grains. Try brown rice instead of white rice, and whole wheat, rye, and corn instead of enriched processed flour. When you eat a lot of whole grains, they replace higher-fat foods in your diet. The B vitamins in whole grains may actually help prevent heart disease, and high-fiber grains help protect against colon cancer.

9. **Switch to fat-free dairy.**
Milk, cheese, cottage cheese, and yogurt are good sources of protein. However, full-fat dairy products are high in saturated fat, so choose fat-free or low-fat varieties. If you have difficulty digesting the lactose contained in dairy products, you can eliminate them from your diet and get your protein from other sources. You can also buy lactose-free dairy products such as Lactaid.

10. Maximize your fiber.

    The health benefits of a high-fiber diet cannot be refuted. You should aim for twenty-five to thirty grams of fiber a day. Most adults eat only half that. To maximize your fiber, eat whole-grain, high-fiber cereals. Top your cereals with fresh fruits or berries. Eat whole-grain bread with at least two grams of fiber per slice. Eat brown or wild rice and whole-grain pastas. Consider adding beans to stews, soups, and casseroles. Eat plenty of fresh and dried fruits.

Ten TriEnergetics Golden Rules for Eating for Dynamic Energy and Better Health

1. Enjoy eating.

2. Eat less.

3. Do not add oils or fats to your food.

4. Eat all of the fruit and vegetables you want.

5. Become more of a vegetarian.

6. Snack with discretion.

7. Fat free does not mean healthy.

8. Eat complex carbohydrates whenever you can.

9. Switch to fat-free dairy.

10. Maximize your fiber.

Moving On

Let's move on now to the next chapter, where we'll discuss the very important issue of what supplements you need to add to your diet to maximize your health.

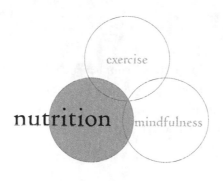

chapter 6

Nature's Weapons Against Aging: Antioxidants Can Help You Stay Younger

A recent study published in a prestigious medical journal demonstrated a pronounced reduction in heart disease in women who consumed high doses of vitamin E. Immediately, another report denounced these findings, claiming vitamin E was ineffectual. A third report supported the first report's findings, but concluded that vitamin E was beneficial only when eaten in foods, not when taken as a capsule. A fourth report contradicted these findings, stating that any natural vitamin E supplement was beneficial, just not the synthetic vitamin E. Following this came a report that synthetic vitamin E was actually harmful and blocked the positive effects of natural vitamin E. Finally, another report concluded that taking vitamin E in any form made no difference whatsoever.

Confusing? You bet. And as more information becomes available, odds are that things are going to get more and more confusing. In the last two years, the once dormant nutritional supplement industry has erupted into a $17.4 billion market. Vitamin companies prey upon the growing concerns of the aging baby boomers, making unproven claims about products and adding vitamins and antioxidants to everything from candy bars to chewing gum and diet soda.

BIASED RESEARCH AND THE ANTIOXIDANT CONTROVERSY

With all the hype building up around this controversial subject, it's easy for you, the consumer, to be taken for a ride. You can look to scientific reports to get accurate information on the benefits of antioxidants, but scientific studies can be designed or interpreted to support just about any reasonable conclusion. Researchers can do this by approaching the data in a particular way or choosing a study group that will be more likely to support a particular conclusion. In medicine, we call this biased research.

There is a tremendous amount of biased research being reported in the popular media from scientists on both sides of the controversy about supplements. Each side claims with absolute conviction that its conclusions are correct. Since the press knows that any controversial health issue will appeal to their audience and increase ratings, they report these findings recklessly and often without regard for scientific accuracy.

You, the consumer, are left to drown in a flood of information, wondering what to do.

DISTILLING THE TRUTH ABOUT ANTIOXIDANTS

The truth is, there is a tremendous amount of healing power in vitamins and antioxidants. There is strong scientific data about free radicals and how they age the body and lead to disease. There's also good scientific data, from nonbiased studies, on the ability of antioxidants and vitamins to stop and even reverse these dangerous aging effects.

This data is so compelling that we have made nutritional supplements an integral part of the TriEnergetics program. In fact, we believe that it's nearly impossible to maintain good health, feel younger, and look better without adding antioxidants and vitamins to your daily routine.

Still, the question remains: how much of the research can you believe? The sheer volume of reports makes it hard to interpret all this data. Some of it is clearly hype, and some of it is clearly biased. Where is the middle ground?

In this chapter, sticking with what has been proven in good, unbiased scientific studies, we will distill the truth about vitamins and antioxidants. We will throw out the chaff and bring you the heart of this very important matter.

UNDERSTANDING FREE RADICALS

> It's a straightforward chemical problem. Free radicals cause damage and antioxidants decrease the damage.
>
> —Denham Harman

Everybody gets older, but does that mean everyone has to age? This question has puzzled scientists and philosophers for years. What is aging? What causes the body to slowly deteriorate and change? What causes the arteries to harden, the skin to slacken, and the immune system to run out of steam? And most importantly, is there anything that can be done to prevent this?

Fortunately, answers are beginning to emerge. Exercise and stress management, two critical elements of the TriEnergetics program, have been shown to be powerful tools in the body's war against aging. However, they are only part of the answer.

In our opinion, the most exciting health discovery since the introduction of antibiotics to cure infection was the discovery of free radicals and the understanding of the role that they play in disease. It was only forty-five years ago that Denham Harman first introduced his unconventional theory that wild molecules whizzed inside the cells, causing damage to the membranes and nuclei. He proposed that it was the accumulative effects of years and years of damage from these molecules that caused the body to age. Dr. Harman called these wild, destructive molecules *free radicals.*

Now, after years of research and thousands upon thousands of scientific experiments by hundreds of researchers, Harman's theory has been shown to be correct.

WHAT ARE FREE RADICALS?

Normally, all molecules in the body maintain a balance of positively charged particles *(protons)* and negatively charged particles *(electrons).* This allows the molecule to be stable and neutral. In the simplest sense, free radicals are molecules that lack one electron, making them unbalanced and active.

You can't avoid free radicals. Breathing, the very process that allows you to live, is also responsible for the creation of these metabolically dangerous chemicals.

OXYGEN: FRIEND OR FOE?

In general, oxygen is considered a good thing. You need oxygen to run your cells, fuel your muscles, and energize your mind. In actuality, oxygen is a very toxic compound, and you can only tolerate it in small amounts.

As you read this, you are breathing air that is 21 percent oxygen. Traveling through your nose and mouth, it enters your lungs and is transported to your bloodstream, where it's delivered to the tissues. Every cell in your body requires this oxygen to fuel its metabolic functions. Once inside the cell, oxygen is metabolized to carbon dioxide and water in a very delicate biochemical process that produces the fuel that runs your cells.

That is where your problems begin. In its conversion to carbon dioxide and water, the oxygen molecule goes through a series of chemical reactions. Unfortunately, these reactions create some very dangerous by-products: electrically charged molecules that lack an electron, or free radicals. Think of them as the body's internal nuclear waste.

THE GREAT ELECTRON HEIST

Everything in nature needs to be in balance, so a molecule that lacks an electron will try to steal one from another molecule to bring itself back in balance. This is exactly what free radicals do. The negatively charged oxygen molecule collides with a cell membrane and steals an electron. This begins a chain reaction. Thousands of free radical reactions occur within seconds as one molecule steals an electron from another. The end result of all this electron swiping is the oxidation of your cell membranes.

Now, you're familiar with the process of oxidation. *Oxidation* is what happens to metal when it's left out in the rain. It becomes rusty. That is exactly what free radicals do to every cell in your body. They devitalize your healthy membranes, turning your young, vital cells into decaying, aging cells, which in turn leads to the decay and aging of your body. Free radicals are turning your cell membranes into the biological equivalent of rusted metal.

RUSTY CELLS ARE DYING CELLS

Once damaged or "rusted," a cell membrane can no longer transport nutrients, oxygen, and water into the cell or remove wastes from the cell. As a result, the cell—a tiny part of you—dies. In some cases, the damage is so severe that the membranes rupture and release their cellular components into the circulation, damaging even more cells in turn.

Free radicals can also act inside a cell by attacking the nucleus of the cell, where the DNA is stored. There, free radicals can steal electrons from the DNA, severely disrupting the DNA strands. This disruption leads to mutations that cause cancer.

In fact, free radicals play a role in causing or exacerbating almost every known disease. Free radicals promote inflammation, which can cause arthritis and skin diseases. They also suppress the immune system, leaving you susceptible to infections and disease. They cause deterioration of tissues, as in macular degeneration of the retina, and they even oxidize fats and cholesterol, causing the clotting process that leads to heart disease.

EXERCISE AND FREE RADICALS

Many people have taken to regular, strenuous exercise to help their bodies stay young. Regular exercise is absolutely vital for total wellness and is an integral part of the TriEnergetics plan, but what do you think happens when you exercise without protecting yourself from free radicals?

When you exercise, your metabolism increases and so does the generation of free radicals. The more you exercise, the more free radicals you make. In all the ways we've just explained, this can be dangerous. Have you ever noticed the number of prominent athletes that die young of heart disease? Some experts believe that this may be caused by an accumulation of free radical damage to the body.

YOU CAN'T ESCAPE THEM

To make matters worse, free radicals aren't only formed inside the body. Free radicals are also caused by exposure to pollution, ozone, and cigarette smoke and are created by radiation. In fact, you are bombarded by billions of free radicals every day.

As a result, you age.

Five Aging Effects of Free Radicals

> oxidation of cell membranes, which leads to cell death

> mutation of DNA, which leads to cancer

> impairment of the immune system, which leads to illness

> oxidation of cholesterol, which leads to heart disease

> deterioration of tissues

IT'S A WAR IN THERE

Normally, your body copes with some of the free radicals you produce by creating special enzymes like *superoxide dismutase* and *glutathione peroxidase*.

These and other powerful enzymes are made by the body specifically to protect against the assault of free radicals on your tissues. But with the constant bombardment of internal and external free radicals, your natural defenses can be quickly overwhelmed, leaving you vulnerable.

When free radicals win the battle, your body suffers the unrelenting effects of aging and disease. But don't worry, help is on the way.

ANTIOXIDANTS: YOUR WEAPONS AGAINST AGING

> People who take antioxidants are physiologically younger and less likely to develop disease.
>
> —Denham Harman

Antioxidants combat the toxic effects of free radicals. They act as scavengers, binding to free radicals and neutralizing them before they can cause damage. By doing so, they slow the process of age-related cell damage.

Five Age-Defying Powers of Antioxidants

› neutralize free radicals

› prevent tissue deterioration

› protect cell membranes

› protect DNA

› enhance immune function

Antioxidants perform these amazing, age-defying feats in one of two ways. Some antioxidants are minerals, such as selenium and zinc, that work in conjunction with the antioxidant enzymes we mentioned earlier. These minerals are necessary for the enzymes to function properly and protect the body from damage. If your diet doesn't supply an adequate amount of these key antioxidant minerals, the enzymes can't do their job and your cells suffer the consequences.

Other nutrients act as antioxidants independent of enzyme systems. Vitamin E and beta carotene mix into the fatty cell membranes and take up position like soldiers on the front line. There, they provide the first line of defense against damage when a free radical comes to attack the membrane. Vitamin E is particularly effective; one vitamin E molecule can disarm up to a thousand free radicals. Vitamin C, which is water soluble, floats around in the bloodstream and body fluids, acting like a roving scout, wiping out free radicals as they march through the body.

Now here's the key. Essential vitamins cannot be manufactured by the body. You must get them from your diet or from supplements.

The standard American diet (SAD) is woefully deficient in antioxidant vitamins and minerals. If you want to maintain an adequate supply of these wellness-preserving compounds in your body, we recommend that you supplement your diet. A healthy supply of antioxidants creates a powerful army of free radical neutralizers in your body.

THE IMMUNE SYSTEM AND NUTRITION

I worry that more than 70 percent of all Americans will die prematurely from diseases caused by or compounded by deficiencies of antioxidants.

—Lester Packer

In the next chapter, which is about stress, we'll discuss the immune system—the body's defense against infection and cancer. A fully functioning immune system is absolutely vital for good health, because the immune system recognizes foreign invaders, bacteria, or cancer cells and destroys them. We'll also point out that stress has a serious detrimental effect on the immune system, increasing your vulnerability to illness.

Poor nutrition can have this same detrimental effect.

Like the rest of your body, the immune system is compromised by an inadequate intake of nutrients. How severely the system is damaged depends on which vitamins or minerals are deficient, but in general, all functions of the immune system are affected by malnutrition. It's been shown that even mild deficiencies of certain nutrients can alter the size and composition of the immune system organs (lymph nodes, spleen, bone marrow, and thymus glands) and can reduce the number of white blood cells in the body. An inadequate intake of one or more vitamins or minerals can wipe out your immune response and set you up for infection and cancer.

Not only that, but when you are under stress, your fight-or-flight hormone cascade is activated, triggering the release of cortisol and catecholamines. These hormones rush through the body, suppressing your immune system, accelerating your metabolism, and increasing your production of free radicals. So stress not only wipes out your immune system, but it also increases your need for antioxidants.

If you are deficient in antioxidants at times of stress, it's only a matter of time before you become ill.

● Sandy's Story: The Visionary Dr. Pauling

I went to one of the top medical schools in the country, Washington University in Saint Louis, and had a wonderful education. My biochemistry class was taught by Nobel laureates Carl and Gerti Cori. In that class, I and my classmates learned a tremendous amount about the chemistry of the human organism, but we learned nothing about nutrition.

Back then, we were taught that the secret to good health was to eat a balanced diet. This would supply all of the nutrition the body needed. We were told that there was absolutely no need to take supplements. I acted accordingly: I tried to eat a balanced diet and turned my nose up at anyone who talked about supplements.

Then several things happened. If you believe in fate, you would say that they weren't coincidental. I was in my first year of residency when a series of respiratory infections knocked me off my feet and put me in the hospital. Even after I was released I had no energy, and I immediately had a relapse of the illness. When I could finally return to work, I was run-down and vulnerable.

One of my professors was working with a famous private patient, two-time Nobel laureate Linus Pauling. The professor told me that Pauling was an amazing man, in wonderful health for his age, who never got ill. Dr. Pauling, my professor learned, took large doses of vitamin C every day and took even more if he was feeling as though he was coming down with something.

At that time, there was absolutely no scientific evidence for taking vitamin C as a supplement unless you had scurvy, which I didn't. But if a man as brilliant as Linus Pauling believed it was helpful, who was I to doubt it? Besides, I was so sick I had nothing to lose.

I started taking two grams of vitamin C a day in divided doses. Within weeks, my health improved dramatically, my respiratory ailment vanished, and my energy skyrocketed. To this day, I take extra vitamin C daily. I believe that vitamin C, working as the primary water-soluble free radical scavenger, helped me to regain my health.

Many people thought Dr. Pauling was an eccentric who went overboard with his vitamin C theory, but as time goes by there is more and more evidence for the beneficial effect of vitamin C. In my mind, Dr. Pauling was a visionary who opened doors to chambers that we are just beginning to explore.

HOW ANTIOXIDANTS BOOST IMMUNITY

Let's take a moment to zero in on how these vital antioxidant vitamins and minerals function to keep your immune system in tip-top shape. And remember, a good immune system doesn't just protect you from infections, it protects against cancer as well.

- Zinc is essential for antibody production, normal thymus function, and the effectiveness of T-lymphocyte helper cells, all of which are vital to fighting infections.

- Iron deficiency impairs lymphocyte activity and causes atrophy of lymphoid tissue, resulting in decreased antibody formation.

- Manganese, magnesium, and selenium strengthen the immune response.

- The B complex vitamins are involved in many aspects of cellular metabolism, and deficiencies in these vitamins weaken resistance and immune response.

- Pyridoxine (vitamin B_6) deficiency causes a loss of lymphoid tissue and depressed antibody responses.

- Deficiencies of pantothenic acid, riboflavin, folic acid, vitamin B_{12}, biotin, thiamine, vitamin A, and vitamin E cause an impaired antibody response.

- Vitamin E, beta carotene, and vitamin C play an essential role in maintaining immune function by preventing free radical damage to immune cells and tissues.

- Even marginal deficiency of vitamin C decreases white cell formation and impairs wound healing.

Quite a wallop from a few vitamins and minerals.

This is why it's so vital to maintain an adequate supply of antioxidants in your body. When you're sick, injured, or under stress, your need for these vitamins will go up, and you must be careful to meet the extra demand.

A WORD OF CAUTION: YOU CAN OVERDO A GOOD THING

It's important to understand that the immune system can be stimulated only to a certain extent with supplements. Beyond this point, larger doses may actually impair the immune response. There is some evidence that vitamin C in doses greater than several grams a day and zinc in doses greater than 150 milligrams per day might interfere with the immune response. There's also evidence that megadoses of some vitamins and minerals may be toxic to the body.

Don't exceed our recommended amounts for any vitamins or minerals.

THE RECOMMENDED DIETARY ALLOWANCES

We hope that by now you realize the potential benefits of supplementing your diet with these powerful compounds. The next question is, how much should you take?

The *recommended dietary allowances* (RDAs) are suggested levels of intake for some of the essential nutrients. These guidelines were established by the Food and Nutrition Board, National Research Council of the National Academy of Sciences. The guidelines are updated about every five years. The RDAs are based on a person's age, sex, weight, and height and are available for

› calories	› vitamin B_6	› vitamin E	› niacin
› protein	› vitamin B_{12}	› folic acid	› phosphorus
› vitamin A	› vitamin C	› iodine	› selenium
› vitamin B_1	› calcium	› vitamin K	› zinc
› vitamin B_2	› vitamin D	› magnesium	

The RDAs are only estimates of nutrient needs; they might be inadequate if, because of long-term illness or poor dietary habits, a person needed to restore depleted vitamin and mineral stores.

Furthermore, the RDAs are based on the nutrient requirements for healthy people to prevent classical nutrient-deficiency diseases. The guidelines don't consider the relationship these nutrients might have to the prevention of other diseases.

Let's rephrase that last point. *The RDA is the least amount of a vitamin you need each day to prevent a specific disease.*

Most vitamins are associated with a classical deficiency disease. The best known of these is *scurvy,* a disease associated with lack of vitamin C and characterized by skin rashes, gum disease, missing teeth, bleeding, anemia, and hemorrhaging. In seafaring days, sailors would spend months at sea, living on a diet of meat, bread, beer, and water. While this diet provided adequate iron and B vitamins, it was almost completely devoid of vitamin C. Sooner or later, the sailors all developed scurvy.

When physicians of the time recognized that the problem was caused by a lack of balance in the sailors' food, they recommended that the sailors bring along supplies of limes, lemons, and other citrus foods. These are all high in vitamin C. Sailors would walk around sucking on limes all day to get their vitamin C. (This is why British sailors came to be known as limeys.) As a result, scurvy became extremely rare amongst the sailors.

The RDAs for vitamin C set by the government represent the least amount that you must ingest daily to prevent scurvy. That's all. There is no consideration of the amount of vitamin C necessary to promote wellness, combat aging, or revitalize your immune system.

To get this information, you would have to turn to the thousands of scientific papers in the medical literature. We have done this research for you and have created the TriEnergetics nutritional supplement program. We'll guide you in using antioxidants, vitamins, and minerals to promote wellness and fight disease.

MUST YOU SUPPLEMENT?

If all these antiaging essential vitamins are present in food, why must you supplement?

You, like us, were probably taught the old paradigm that a balanced diet would supply all of the vitamins and minerals you need. But most people don't eat a balanced diet, they eat the SAD diet. The American Dietetic Association estimates that only one in ten people eat the recommended number of servings of fruits and vegetables. People have increased their consumption of grains, but they are still more likely to eat something made with refined flour than with whole grains.

In the average American diet, 59 percent of the calories come from nutrient-poor food sources. In fact, the food is so nutritionally depleted that most Americans are on the verge of serious vitamin deficiencies. This is a major problem. A huge number of American adults—especially older adults—are well below the bare minimum of daily vitamin intake.

The issue goes far beyond just meeting the RDAs. If you meet the RDA of a particular nutrient, you can be certain that you will not develop a deficiency disease, but that doesn't mean that you have enough of that nutrient—especially the antioxidants—to help prevent chronic diseases, cancers, and age-related diseases.

The bottom line is that there is no way to get enough antioxidants to effectively retard aging from food alone. Vitamin E is a prime example. In order to get the optimal daily dose of vitamin E, you would have to eat 5,000 to 20,000 calories a day, nearly all fat!

SUPPLEMENTING SENSIBLY

We recommend a well-balanced multiple vitamin and mineral supplement for everyone. We also suggest that you increase the amount of vitamin C beyond the basic level when you're ill or under stress.

Be very cautious about taking megadoses of supplements. The fat-soluble vitamins (A, D, and K) accumulate in the tissues and have known toxic effects. Large doses of iron can interfere with zinc absorption, and large doses of zinc can suppress immune function. Some of the B vitamins can also have toxic effects when taken in large doses. Vitamin E in doses greater than 200 IU may not be safe.

Due to potential toxic effects of certain vitamins and minerals in high concentrations, you should take no more than three times the RDA for any of the supplements.

Here are the TriEnergetics recommendations for the optimal daily intake of essential nutrients and antioxidants.

vitamin A	25,000 IU
beta carotene	25,000 IU
vitamin D	400 IU
vitamin E	200 IU
vitamin B_1	25 mg
vitamin B_2	25 mg
niacin	25 mg
vitamin B_6	50 mg
vitamin B_{12}	20 μg
folic acid	400 μg
pantothenic acid	10 mg
vitamin C	1,000 mg
calcium	400 mg
chromium	100 μg
copper	3 mg
iron	
none for men	
postmenopausal women	10 mg
premenopausal women	25 mg
magnesium	200 mg
manganese	5 mg
selenium	200 μg
zinc	15 mg
coenzyme Q_{10}	90 mg
grape seed extract	100 mg
citrus bioflavonoids	1,000 mg
alpha-lipoic acid	100 mg
glutathione	100 mg

Moving On

Now let's move ahead and look at the next important approach to maintaining your health: learning how to manage your stress.

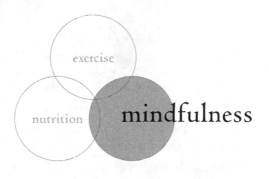

chapter 7

The Dragon Within: The Deadly Physiology of Stress

> It does not do to leave a dragon out of your calculations, if you live near him.
>
> —J. R. R. Tolkien

Stress!

In our fast-paced society, stress is everywhere. It's the deadly dragon within you, breathing fire into your body, tearing you apart. It's as pervasive as oxygen or water. E-mail, cell phones, traffic, bills, children, bosses: the onslaught never ends.

Stress!

Sound familiar? We bet it does. People run around so much of the time, hurrying here, rushing there, honking their horns, swearing at other drivers on the freeway, trying to meet a deadline or get the kids to practice on time.

Stress!

Most people don't even take the time to sit down to eat a meal any more. Fast-food restaurants are making a killing (literally, given the quality of the food they serve) designing and packaging food to be more convenient for the commuter generation. One fast-food chain developed a hamburger shaped like a hot dog so that commuting women could eat it while driving without spilling the contents all over their blouses. And they call this progress!

STRESS IS ONLY GETTING WORSE

As life becomes increasingly complicated, with more pressures and more demands coming from jobs, finances, and relationships, people's level of stress will continue to skyrocket. In fact, many of our patients report feeling stressed out at least once a week.

The latest boom in high-tech information systems is only further contributing to the stress. Just look around you. How many people do you see conducting business over cell phones, frantically reading and sending e-mail, or finishing last-minute projects on laptops?

Stress has expanded beyond the workplace and escaped the confines of the nine-to-five job to invade every aspect of daily life.

Did you know that some studies suggest that over 60 percent of all traffic accidents are the result of road rage or overly aggressive driving? Fifteen years ago, the term "road rage" hadn't even been invented; now it is talked about as if it is some naturally occurring disease that needs research, studies, drugs, and treatment.

Road rage is not a disease, it is a symptom. The disease is stress, and stress kills.

MORE STRESS, LESS FUN

The sad thing is that as career demands increase, the first thing to suffer is leisure time and relaxation. The very thing needed to combat the stress is the first thing to get pushed farther and farther down the priority list. People rarely take the time to detoxify the stress that rampages through their bodies.

It's no wonder that stress is killing people.

The Typical American Success Story

One of our associates in the medical business ran a very busy practice. He was quite successful, the envy of his peers. He split his time among three offices, commuting from one to another several times a day. Surgery? On Thursday? That must have been in city A. Office time on Tuesday? Morning or afternoon? Oh yes, that must have been in city B.

This hectic pace—combined with the day-to-day stress of running a business, marketing, billing, hiring, and firing—was like a dragon, slowly eating away at him, burning a hole through his belly. It was no surprise to any of us when he was admitted to the hospital for treatment of a bleeding ulcer.

Stress had literally eaten a hole through him.

Does this sound familiar to you? Maybe it's not working in three different offices that's getting to you; maybe it's trying to get three kids to three different places at the same time. Maybe it's three different work projects stacking up on your desk, or three extra bills draining your bank account.

Whatever it is, you'd better believe that stress affects everyone, including you.

STRESS CAUSES ILLNESS

Sure, stress is unpleasant, but is it really a health problem? The answer is a definite yes. Stress is a major cause of illness and has been implicated as one of the most important factors responsible for a whole host of diseases. Let's look at one particularly awful example.

MONDAY MORNING HEART ATTACKS

If you are like most people, the last thing you want to hear after a relaxing Sunday is that alarm going off at 6:00 A.M. on Monday. Sometimes, if you know that you have a particularly busy day ahead of you, you can feel the stress even before the alarm sounds. Your mind will race as you think about everything that you have to do the next day—where you need to go, who you need to meet, and what you need to accomplish. Your sleep is ruined by worry. Oftentimes, you wake up before the alarm goes off, feeling tired and weak as though you hadn't slept at all.

Can you relate to this?

Many people are stressed when they go back to work after a weekend off. But can this type of stress affect your health? It sure can. In fact, a study found that the incidence of heart attacks among the European workforce increased by 33 percent on Mondays (Friedman 1994). Monday morning stress causes Monday morning heart attacks.

There's no doubt about it—stress kills.

STRESS AND COPING

Everyone feels stress. The real question is, can you do anything about it? Absolutely. How you deal with stress has a serious impact on both your psychological and physical health.

But let's face it. Most people don't have the skills to handle stress well. After all, where were you supposed to have learned these skills? In school? You learned math, English, and history. Maybe you even got a little sex education. But we bet you were never taught in school how to recognize and relieve stress.

DENIAL, DENIAL, DENIAL

The honest truth is that most people don't ever learn to cope with stress. When it comes to stress management, the average adult knows next to nothing. The most commonly used method of stress management in America is denial. Just ignore the stress and hope it'll go away.

You may fool others into thinking that you are a cool cat who isn't bothered by stress, but you can't fool your body. When you're under stress, your blood pressure will go up, your pulse will quicken, you'll breathe faster, and free radicals will bombard your cells.

We call this stress *mis*management, because denial doesn't effectively protect your body against the ravages of stress. If you are stressed your body will know it, and in the end you will be the loser.

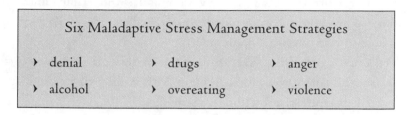

Six Maladaptive Stress Management Strategies

› denial	› drugs	› anger
› alcohol	› overeating	› violence

Imagine if our country's foreign policy during World War II had been *ignore it and it will go away*. Clearly, the war would have had a different outcome. The same can be said about your war against stress. You can't treat stress by pretending it isn't there. The stress doesn't just go away; it stays with you, and ignoring it can have serious long-term effects on your health.

WHAT IS STRESS?

Before we discuss the mechanisms by which stress causes illness, let's take a moment to consider the biological definition of stress.

Stress Defined

Stress is any external or internal stimulation that causes a physiologic reaction in an organism.

According to this definition, stress is everywhere. Walking is stress on the muscles; it causes the muscles to work harder, to burn energy, and to make more muscle tissue. Eating is stress on the digestive system; it causes the release of digestive enzymes, it alters blood flow so more blood rushes to the intestines to absorb nutrients, and it stimulates peristalsis. All of these are physiologic reactions to a stimulus.

107

But stress can come from anywhere. Stress can come from your work, your neighbors, your children, or even your own mind. Each of these stressors can cause a physiologic reaction in your body. When you're overwhelmed at work, your heart will beat faster, your muscles will clamp down, your digestion will be upset, and your blood pressure will skyrocket. Each of these is a physiologic reaction to a stimulus.

You can't avoid stress. Every organism on this planet is susceptible. Even an amoeba experiences stress. Poke it with a micropipette, and it will move away. This is stress: a reaction to a stimulus.

WHY YOU NEED STRESS

The reason stress exists is that in many ways, stress is both necessary and beneficial to life. Stress helps animals grow and adapt. It stimulates change. It helps an animal to escape predators. It guides plants to grow toward the sunshine. It helps guide that poor amoeba toward food and away from harm.

In humans, stress stimulates the muscles to grow after exercise. It drives us to eat and drink when the needs arise. It guides us away from danger.

STRESS IS SUBJECTIVE

While stress may be a universal constant, the way each individual reacts to stress is distinctly personal. You form your own reaction to a stimulus, whether it be walking, eating, or your boss yelling at you. Your own unique personality, behaviors, and coping skills determine how you react to that stimulus.

So then, for the purposes of this book, let's offer another definition of stress.

The TriEnergetics Definition of Stress

Stress is a subjective experience consisting of a situation, your perception of the situation, and your reaction to that situation.

Given this definition, you can see that what is stressful to one person may be inconsequential to another. Some people are incredibly stressed by speaking in public, others do it without a moment's thought. Work deadlines affect some people more than others. It's a very individual thing.

Todd's Tale: Horror in the Research Lab

As a young behavioral biology student, I spent a great amount of time in the physiologic psychology laboratory, searching to understand human behavior. When I was working on my thesis, I had the unsavory job of assisting one of my professors in her research, which involved rats, alcohol, and tobacco.

The premise was simple. To see whether there was a relationship between nicotine, stress, and alcohol consumption, we implanted nicotine pellets under the skin of several large white rats. After a stressful stimulation, the rats were given a choice of drinking from a bottle containing water or one containing alcohol, and we measured how much alcohol the rats consumed.

The problem was how to stress the rats. And that's where I came in.

Now, you must understand, if I could have simply imposed some sort of work deadline on the rats, I would have. I would have let them drive in traffic, get yelled at by my boss—I would even have let them pay my bills. But let's face it, that wouldn't work on a rat.

No. In scientific circles, the way to stress rats is to put them in a cage that has an electrified floor and deliver an electric shock to their feet every five seconds for five minutes.

Stressful? You bet. But you know what? It was more stressful for me than for the rats. I couldn't stand pulling them out of their cages (you can bet they were never too happy to see me) putting them in the electric box, turning it on, and hearing them squeal every five seconds for five minutes. It tore me apart. I even started to have dreams about rats in electric boxes chasing me through the science building.

After the experiment ended, we calculated the rats' alcohol consumption, and it did go up, but you know what? So did mine. The entire time I was doing that research, I was drinking like a fish. I nearly doubled my alcohol intake as an unconscious way of coping with the stress of that experiment.

That situation was extremely stressful for me, yet it might not even have fazed other people. Some of my colleagues have done animal research for years and continue to do it without any stress whatsoever. Not me. If I even see a research cage, my heart picks up a notch and my palms begin to sweat.

Each person has their own individual stress threshold. When that threshold is reached, regardless of how little or how much stimulation it takes to reach it, the stressful effects are felt by the mind and the body.

STRESS: THE GREAT MASQUERADER

In an article published by *Prevention* magazine, 11,000 readers were polled on their perception of how stress affected their lives. Of those readers, 74 percent responded that stress affected their enjoyment of life, and 55 percent responded that they thought stress affected their health.

The signs and symptoms of chronic stress can present themselves in some very subtle ways. You may appear completely calm and cool on the outside while stress is ravaging your body from the inside.

Do you feel tired even though you've supposedly had a good night's sleep? Do you get headaches, or tightness in the neck and shoulders? Do you suffer from constipation or heartburn? These are warning signs that stress is catching up with you.

EXERCISE: Identify Your Stress Symptoms

This exercise looks at problems you may have because of your stress. Take the quiz and see where you fit on the stress scale. You might be surprised.

For each of the symptoms below, check yes, occasionally, or no. Give yourself two points for each yes, one point for each occasionally, and zero points for a no.

Do you suffer from the following?

fatigue	☐ yes	☐ occasionally	☐ no
difficulty falling asleep or staying asleep	☐ yes	☐ occasionally	☐ no
cold sweats	☐ yes	☐ occasionally	☐ no
shallow, rapid breathing	☐ yes	☐ occasionally	☐ no
quick pulse	☐ yes	☐ occasionally	☐ no
chest pains or palpitations	☐ yes	☐ occasionally	☐ no
decreased interest in sex	☐ yes	☐ occasionally	☐ no
indigestion, constipation, diarrhea, or abdominal pain	☐ yes	☐ occasionally	☐ no
muscle tension in the jaw, neck, shoulders, and chest	☐ yes	☐ occasionally	☐ no
teeth grinding	☐ yes	☐ occasionally	☐ no
chronic or frequent headaches	☐ yes	☐ occasionally	☐ no
forgetfulness or inability to concentrate	☐ yes	☐ occasionally	☐ no
physical weakness and exhaustion	☐ yes	☐ occasionally	☐ no
skin rashes	☐ yes	☐ occasionally	☐ no
change in appetite (either overeating or loss of appetite)	☐ yes	☐ occasionally	☐ no
menstrual irregularities	☐ yes	☐ occasionally	☐ no
short temper or impatience	☐ yes	☐ occasionally	☐ no
irrational fears or phobias	☐ yes	☐ occasionally	☐ no
depression	☐ yes	☐ occasionally	☐ no
excessive drinking	☐ yes	☐ occasionally	☐ no
overspending	☐ yes	☐ occasionally	☐ no

Total score: _____

None of these symptoms or problems should be considered normal; however, any of them can occur briefly at times. If you experience any of the above conditions chronically, you may be suffering from a stress-related illness. If you scored higher than two points, stress is probably affecting your health to some degree. If you scored higher than five points, then stress may be playing a large role in your health and you are at risk of developing a serious stress-related illness.

These symptoms, although extremely important, are only the tip of the iceberg. Chronic stress, or acute stress that isn't managed well, can lead to an increased susceptibility to viral and bacterial illness, as well as to the development of chronic diseases such as hypertension, atherosclerosis, and cancer.

Cancer? Come on. Stress is bad, but can it cause cancer?

You bet it can, and later in this chapter, we're going to show you how.

WHO, ME? STRESSED?

Most people, when they think about stress, generally associate it with some pretty nasty experiences: difficult bosses, deadlines, pressure at work. But that's not all. Remember, stress is any experience that causes a physiologic reaction in an organism. Not all stress comes from the workplace.

It's no coincidence that illness often accompanies life changes. How many people you know have become ill in the middle of a family crisis, such as a divorce or death of a loved one? Has this ever happened to you?

Acute life changes can have a tremendous impact on your stress level, and they often go unrecognized. To find the obvious and not-so-obvious stress in your life, take the following quiz.

EXERCISE: Find the Hidden Stress in Your Life

Answer the following questions by checking yes or no. For each yes, give yourself the allotted number of points, then add up the points for your total.

In the last six months:

Has your spouse or partner died?	☐ yes ☐ no	20 points
Have you divorced or separated from your spouse or partner?	☐ yes ☐ no	15 points
Has a close relative died?	☐ yes ☐ no	13 points
Have you been hospitalized or suffered a major illness?	☐ yes ☐ no	11 points
Have you married?	☐ yes ☐ no	10 points
Have you found out you were soon to become a parent?	☐ yes ☐ no	9 points
Has there been an illness in the family?	☐ yes ☐ no	9 points
Have you lost your job or retired?	☐ yes ☐ no	9 points
Are you having stress at work?	☐ yes ☐ no	8 points
Are you having sexual difficulties?	☐ yes ☐ no	8 points
Has a new member been born or married into your family?	☐ yes ☐ no	8 points
Has a close friend died?	☐ yes ☐ no	8 points
Have your finances become better or worse?	☐ yes ☐ no	8 points
Have you changed jobs?	☐ yes ☐ no	8 points
Have any children moved out of the home?	☐ yes ☐ no	6 points
Is trouble with in-laws causing difficulty in your family?	☐ yes ☐ no	6 points
Is there anyone at home or work that you dislike strongly?	☐ yes ☐ no	6 points
Do you travel frequently for work?	☐ yes ☐ no	6 points
Do you frequently have premenstrual tension?	☐ yes ☐ no	6 points

Have you had an important personal success (such as a job promotion)?	☐ yes ☐ no	6 points
Have you had jet leg at least twice in the last two months?	☐ yes ☐ no	6 points
Have you had a major domestic upheaval such as moving or remodeling your home?	☐ yes ☐ no	5 points
Have you had problems at work that may be putting your job at risk?	☐ yes ☐ no	5 points
Have you taken on a large debt or mortgage?	☐ yes ☐ no	3 points
Does your daily commute involve gridlock traffic or long waits for trains or buses?	☐ yes ☐ no	2 points
Have you had a minor brush with the law (such as a traffic violation)?	☐ yes ☐ no	2 points

Total score: _____

The higher your score, the more stressful your life. As a general guide, a score under five suggests that you are not very likely to have a stress-related illness. If your score is fifteen or higher, the pressures on you are substantial. This means you are at a higher risk for stress-related illnesses. As you can see from this quiz, you may not even be aware of some of the stressors that affect your life.

GOOD EVENTS CAN BE STRESSFUL TOO

Not everything that causes you stress is unpleasant. Getting married or getting promoted at work are generally seen as good experiences, yet the sudden change in lifestyle can still have a serious impact on your body.

● Todd's Tale: Wedding Day Bliss

Getting married was one of the most wonderful things that ever happened to me. The wedding went flawlessly at a beautiful location overlooking the Pacific Ocean. Everything flowed smoothly. The cake was delicious, the musicians arrived on time, the weather was perfect.

So why was I completely exhausted when it was over?

Because the wedding, although wonderful, was stressful as all get-out. The planning, the orchestrating, the worrying over details, the decision making, the arranging of rooms for out-of-town guests—plus standing in front of the whole world, declaring your love and praying that nothing goes wrong—that's stress!

It's amazing that any of us live long enough to get through the planning stages and actually get married.

Do you know someone who got sick just before her wedding? After all the planning and preparing, the one thing she didn't bet on was a last-minute case of the flu or laryngitis or even a cold.

It's no coincidence that these illnesses plague you at the least opportune times—before a big presentation or a speech or an important meeting. Stress battles your immune system into submission and invites predatory viruses to sneak up on you when you can least afford to be sick.

HOW STRESS LEADS TO DISEASE

Let's look at the physiology of how stress can actually lead to disease.

FIGHT OR FLIGHT

For centuries, Taoist physicians have recognized the health risks of a stressful lifestyle, but it's only recently that Western scientists have begun to unravel the mystery of how stress affects the body.

The first important work on this subject was done by physiologist Walter Cannon, who described a primitive biological response for survival shared by all animals, including humans. He called this the *fight-or-flight* response and described the changes that it causes in the body.

When confronted with danger, the response of an animal is an increase in blood pressure, an increase in heart rate, and an increase in blood flow to the muscles. This response provides an extra surge of strength and energy to enable the endangered animal to fight for its life or to escape from a predator.

Predators are no longer the main survival concern for humans, but the fight-or-flight response still exists. With each stressor that you encounter, whether a boss, a spouse, or financial pressure, the fight-or-flight response kicks in, driving up your blood pressure and your heart rate.

When you consider the daily bombardment of stressful situations that you encounter, you can see that this response can be in effect nearly the entire day.

THE STRESS CASCADE

The next important contribution in understanding the effect of stress on the body was made by Hans Selye, a celebrated biochemist, who analyzed the physiological changes of the fight-or-flight reaction and discovered that stress leads to a cascade release of hormones in the body.

This cascade is initiated in the *hypothalamus,* a small gland located in the primitive area of the brain. This important gland has exclusive control over the body's most basic functions; it regulates hunger, thirst, sexual function, and body temperature. It effects most of this control by sending signals, in the form of specific neurohormones, to the *pituitary gland.* The pituitary, located at the base of the brain, is the master gland of the endocrine system.

Under times of stress, such as during the fight-or-flight response, the hypothalamus signals the pituitary, which then secretes *adrenocorticotropin* (ACTH). ACTH travels to the *adrenal glands* (which are just above the kidneys) and causes the *adrenal cortex* to pump out a group of hormones referred to as *corticosteroids,* including *cortisol.*

THE HARMFUL EFFECTS OF CORTICOSTEROIDS

Corticosteroids have numerous effects on the body, some beneficial and others harmful. For example, they reduce inflammation in the body, but they also increase blood pressure, cause retention of fluid, and perhaps most importantly suppress immunity.

Corticosteroids Compromise Immunity

Let's put that last statement another way to illustrate what we're talking about. Some of the most powerful medicines we doctors have to combat inflammation—whether from arthritis, autoimmune disease, or asthma—are steroids. Not get-big-muscles steroids, but corticosteroids. These medicines have names like prednisone, cortisone, and dexamethasone, and what they do is stop the body's immune system.

When you are under stress, your own body produces loads and loads of corticosteroids, namely cortisol. Those steroids travel through your veins and stop your immune system. They stop your ability to fight disease. They stop the ability of your white blood cells to accumulate and eat up invading bacteria. They stop the ability of your white cells to proliferate and ward off infection.

When you have high levels of circulating corticosteroids, your defenses are down. You will get sick.

Corticosteroids Contribute to Diabetes

But there's more. Steroids also cause the body to break down lean tissue to boost blood sugar levels. This is essential to supply the muscles with the sugar they need to perform at peak levels in times of danger.

There's a name for chronically elevated blood sugar. It's diabetes, and it is one of the leading health problems in this country. It causes the malfunction of every organ in your body, from your heart to your kidneys to your eyes. It blocks off the blood flow to your legs, sometimes leading to amputations. It decimates your nervous system.

It can kill you. And it may in part be caused by chronic stress and prolonged elevated levels of your own corticosteroids.

Guess what? There's more.

Corticosteroids Make You Vulnerable to Cancer

You have a natural defense against cancer: your immune system. Specifically, your immune system scans certain proteins on your cell walls and reads the proteins like information in a computer file. If the immune system finds the proper encoding of proteins, it recognizes the cell as normal and leaves it alone. If it finds the wrong protein message on the cell, it destroys it.

There are cells in the immune system called *natural killer cells.* The sole purpose of these cells is to scavenge the body, scanning cells for the proper protein sequence and destroying the cells that don't match up. This is your natural defense against cancer. When that cancer cell puts up the wrong protein message, Pow! It gets eaten.

But guess what? Steroids inhibit the scavenging function of natural killer cells. Stress weakens your body's natural ability to ward off cancer. Is it any wonder that cancer rates are constantly on the rise in our stressed-out society?

Corticosteroids Cause Autoimmune Problems

There is a whole host of diseases, called *autoimmune diseases,* in which the body's immune system loses its ability to distinguish the good cells from the bad cells. The immune system then goes about destroying perfectly normal cells because it can't tell the difference between normal cells and bad ones. The result is that your own immune system attacks you. Lupus is one of the better known diseases of this type, but there are many others.

The rates of autoimmune disease are increasing in this country. By now, you can guess the reason: stress.

Stress-induced increases in corticosteroids cause

- decreased immune function
- decreased natural killer cell function
- increased blood sugar
- increased risk of disease
- breakdown of muscle to supply blood sugar
- increased risk of infection
- increased risk of cancer

THE HARMFUL EFFECTS OF CATECHOLAMINES

Clearly, your body suffers when stress triggers a flood of corticosteroids, which are secreted from the cortex of the adrenal glands. But the adrenal gland has a second anatomic part, the inner portion or *adrenal medulla,* and the hypothalamus has a direct impact on that structure as well.

The medulla also manufactures stress hormones. These are the *catecholamines,* the most important of which are epinephrine (also called *adrenaline*) and norepinephrine.

Epinephrine makes the heart beat faster, quickens breathing, and redirects blood flow from your internal organs to the brain and skeletal muscles. *Norepinephrine* increases the rate of breathing and causes a rise in blood pressure by constricting the small blood vessels. These changes are key to the fight-or-flight response. They prepare the animal to fend off an attacker or flee out of harm's way.

Catecholamines Contribute to Heart Disease

All of these responses are useful and important for a gazelle on the African prairie when she sees a lion approach, but what do you think happens to you—a modern human—when you are under constant stress? You have chronically high levels of circulating catecholamines buzzing around in your body, driving up your blood pressure and forcing your heart to pound like a jackhammer. As you sit there and stew in a nasty traffic jam, your catecholamine levels are through the roof.

Coffee only makes the problem worse. Caffeine increases your catecholamine levels, thereby producing the well-known coffee buzz. Given that Americans seem to be addicted to both stress and caffeine, is it any wonder that heart disease is the leading cause of death in the United States?

Catecholamines Cause Other Problems

Catecholamines have other actions also. They stop your digestive system (causing indigestion, diarrhea, and constipation) and get you wired and edgy, moody, angry, maybe even violent. They can make you quick to jump all over someone who cuts you off on the freeway or who fails to respond to your signaled attempts to change lanes.

There's the cause of road rage.

It's also probable that the stress-induced production of catecholamines increases your risk of infectious disease and cancer by impairing the proliferation of *lymphocytes* (a type of white blood cell) in the body and by increasing the number of *T-suppressor cells* (which decrease the immune response). Both of these effects damage your immune defenses.

Stress-induced increases in catecholamines cause	
› increased heart rate	› increased risk of heart disease
› increased blood pressure	
› increased risk of damage to delicate blood vessels	› increased risk of stroke
	› problems with digestion
› increased respiratory rate	› moodiness and anger
› decreased immune system function	› increased risk of infections
	› increased risk of disease

Sounds pretty bad, doesn't it? Well, there's another important way stress can harm you.

120

STRESS HORMONES RELEASE FREE RADICALS

Corticosteroids and catecholamines also serve to crank up your metabolism, causing an increased consumption of oxygen and the production of more free radicals. As you learned in chapter 6, these free radicals circulate through the body, attacking cell membranes and causing cellular damage. This damage adds up to premature aging, illness, and eventually death.

LINKS BETWEEN MIND, BODY, AND IMMUNITY

The discovery of the effects of stress on the immune system has been a milestone in understanding how stress causes disease. For thousands of years, the Taoist sages have written about the mind-body connection. They knew that calmness of mind was necessary for calmness of body. Again, modern science has only recently caught up with the wisdom of the ancients and begun to shed some light on the complex interaction between mind and body.

The scientific discipline that studies this interaction is *psychoneuroimmunology* (PNI). This ungainly word is more easily understood if divided into its three components: *psycho* (the mind), *neuro* (the nervous system) and *immuno* (the immune system). Researchers in this field study the connections between the mind, central nervous system, and immune responses. Research in the field of PNI often involves hormones, because hormones play a major role in linking these three systems.

ONE BODY, ONE MIND

In 1990, investigators in PNI made a major discovery that has revolutionized our approach to medicine. They found that contrary to former belief, the immune system does not act alone, independently of other biological systems in the body. Rather, the immune system is regulated by the brain, by the nervous system, and also by hormones produced by the endocrine system.

This means that you have an interlocking network of biological systems making up your whole person. Your attitudes, emotions, and sensations, as well as your regulation of internal balance and your ability to destroy invading organisms, are subtly but directly interrelated. You experience and respond to stimuli on many levels at once, and all of these levels affect each other. What you feel as an emotion has a profound effect on the way your endocrine and immune systems function.

George Solomon, a professor of psychiatry at University of California, Los Angeles, has identified a number of links between the immune system and the central nervous system:

- Stress can alter a person's immune system.

- Personality characteristics affect the way a person's immune system is influenced by the environment.

- Emotional upset affects the immune system and the incidence, severity, and course of illnesses such as infections and cancer.

- Hormones regulated by the central nervous system influence the immune system.

- Substances produced by the immune system affect the central nervous system.

- Behavioral interventions—such as biofeedback, imagery, and relaxation techniques—enhance immune function.

What this tells us is that chronic stress can have a long-term effect not only on your blood pressure and heart rate but on the function of your immune and endocrine systems as well. Any disruption of the normal immune balance of the body can lead to disease—not just colds and infections but serious diseases, including cancer.

• Todd's Tale: The Blind Artist

Here's a great example of how the mind can affect the health of the body. Frederick came into my office one day, and he was as scared as a turkey the night before Thanksgiving. A successful graphic designer, Frederick was just completing his final project for his master's degree in fine arts when he suddenly went blind in his right eye. He could still see lights, but shapes were blurred and distorted. Needless to say, Frederick panicked.

After I examined him, it became apparent that Frederick had central serous retinopathy (CSR), a visually disabling swelling of the central part of the retina. What makes this disease so interesting is that it has been irrefutably connected to stress. CSR usually happens to young men who have high blood pressure and a type A personality. This description fit Frederick to a T. By his own admission, he was a bubbling cauldron of stress.

It's widely accepted that CSR is caused by high circulating levels of catecholamines triggered by chronic stress. These catecholamines damage the delicate blood vessels of the retina, and as a result, the blood vessels leak serous fluid and the retina swells.

After discussing the situation with Frederick, I talked at length about how stress literally caused him to go blind in one eye, but I reassured him that the blindness would resolve if he could make adjustments in his lifestyle.

Frederick began changing his life, using the exercises I gave him to cool down his stress. The change was dramatic. At his follow-up visit, six weeks later, not only was Frederick more relaxed and calm, but his vision had improved dramatically.

MIND OVER MATTER: STRESS MANAGEMENT IS ESSENTIAL

We now know that mind and health are so intimately connected that many diseases formerly thought to be either purely mental or purely physical are now seen to be an interaction of both.

Two conclusions are inevitable:

- The mind has powers over the body that few Westerners thought possible.

- Stress is the dragon within, and it can cause a person to become profoundly ill.

In light of this, you can see that it is absolutely essential to develop healthy techniques for managing the stress in your life.

123

Moving On

Let's move on to the next chapter and see how to do just that.

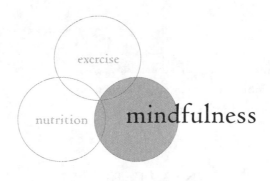

chapter 8

Taming the Dragon: How to Become Healthier by Sitting Quietly and Doing Nothing

> The reason that worry kills more people than work is that more people worry than work.
>
> —Robert Frost

In every travel agency, you'll see the same thing. On the wall there's a huge poster of a faraway place where the beaches are white, the water is blue, and life is perfect. There may be a hammock and a drink with a pink umbrella. The scene is amazingly tranquil. Perhaps, at one time or another, you have looked longingly at that scene and wished that you were there, relaxing in the hammock, soaking in the sun, leaving your worries behind.

Unfortunately, if you're like most people, you usually don't have the time or money to get away, and when you do, your worries come along with you like unwanted baggage.

STRESS IS INEVITABLE

Worry is built into the American way of life.

You're bombarded daily with problems and stressful situations. Each problem and every situation brings with it the potential for stress. The greater and more prolonged the stress, the more likely it is that your health will suffer.

You can't escape it. Stress is part of your everyday life, as common as oxygen or water. So, since you can't avoid it, you may as well learn how to deal with it.

YOUR STRESS THRESHOLD VARIES

We bet that like most people, you have good days and bad days. On the good days, you are strong and even-keeled. On the bad days, you feel as though you are wallowing in the muck and can't get it together. On the good days, you're more resistant to stress. On the bad days, you're an easy mark.

Have you ever wondered why you are more likely to get stressed on the bad days? It's because on bad days, your stress threshold is lower and you're more vulnerable. On good days, your stress threshold is higher and you're more resistant. It all comes down to how much stress you can tolerate at a given moment.

The *stress threshold* is the amount of stress you can handle before you develop symptoms. It varies from day to day and sometimes from minute to minute. On one occasion you can be exposed to many stressful situations without ill effect, while on another it may take only one worry or one problem to overwhelm you.

Your stress threshold is determined by everything that has happened to you in the past, by how you feel at the moment, and by what else has happened to you during that day. The threshold is completely dependent upon your mental, emotional, and physical state at that moment.

In order to have more resistance to stress, you need to raise your threshold.

> Your stress threshold is the amount of stress that you can handle on any given day without untoward mental and physical health effects.

SERENITY RAISES YOUR STRESS THRESHOLD

The key to mastering stress and raising your threshold is to gain serenity.

Horns honking! Traffic jams! Kids screaming! Bosses yelling! Flight delays! Road rage! The frantic pace of Western life throws one obstacle after another in your way. Serenity is as incompatible to the Western lifestyle as truth is to politicians.

But it doesn't have to be that way. In the Far East, serenity has been studied for thousands of years. There, it is cherished as a virtue. Entire schools of thought are devoted to finding ways of becoming serene.

We have taken the best of these practices for developing serenity and incorporated them into the TriEnergetics program. In the following pages, we'll show you how you can use these techniques to develop serenity. These techniques are simple to learn and will fit comfortably into your lifestyle. They'll help you battle stress, strengthen your body's natural immune defenses, and improve your health. These techniques will help you get through stressful situations with ease and grace.

SIT STILL AND DO NOTHING

The cornerstone of the TriEnergetics stress management program is a very simple, easy practice that you've already heard of: meditation.

We realize that you may already have an image of what meditation means. You may picture a swami sitting on an isolated mountaintop. Or you may picture an aging hippie in a tie-dyed T-shirt sitting surrounded by burning incense.

While these images may be true in certain instances, meditation is not only or even primarily an act of the counterculture. The truth is, meditation is a powerful, scientifically based medical tool. A significant amount of good, nonbiased research has verified the benefits of regular meditation:

- reduced heart rate

- relaxed blood vessels

- lowered blood pressure

- reduced breathing rate

- reduced oxygen intake

- decreased sweating

- reduced anxiety

- improved relaxation

- improved digestion

- enhanced immune response

These claims have been proven with solid medical research. Not only that, but people who have worked through the meditation portion of our program have reported that their mind is quieter and that they're less agitated by emotional setbacks. Those with high blood pressure found that their blood pressure lowered significantly. Those with anxieties found relief. Those with worries found peace.

This can happen for you, too!

Sandy's Story: The Meditation Revelation

I began the practice of meditation in the 1970s after my wife and I attended a lecture on Transcendental Meditation in Berkeley, California. We attended the lecture mostly out of curiosity, but what the speakers said hooked us immediately.

What caught my attention in particular were references to the work done by Herbert Benson, a cardiologist at Harvard Medical School. Dr. Benson studied people who had a regular practice of meditation and found that they lowered their blood pressure, pulse rate, and basal metabolic rate when they meditated. It was remarkable to me that so much could be accomplished by doing so little—literally by sitting and doing nothing.

I was a skeptic, but I signed up for the training. I learned that meditation was a process of focused relaxation. In the Transcendental Meditation training we were each given a mantra, which we were told was our own unique, private, and very special sound that we were to use when meditating. We were told that we should never tell our mantra to any other living soul. Armed with my magical mantra, I delved into the meditation practice. Within a few weeks of meditating, I noticed a remarkable effect. My blood pressure, previously moderately high, had decreased to a normal level. Events that used to either threaten or stress me no longer bothered me. My life seemed to run on a more even keel.

I was very excited about this transformation. Most of my classmates were as well. Once the training was completed, many of us revealed our mantras to each other as a way of sharing our good fortune. That was when we made a shocking discovery. The mantras the instructors had given us were not unique. Many people had the exact same mantra.

After learning this, some people thought they'd been cheated, and quite a few became discouraged and quit meditating.

Not me. The revelation had the opposite effect on me. I realized that there is nothing mystical or magical about meditation. No special mantras are needed. Meditation is merely a time of focused relaxation, a technique that anyone can use to combat the stress of daily life.

GETTING STARTED

Everyone has the need for a time of inner peace. Carry out the meditation daily and you will see amazing results. The beneficial effects of simply relaxing are so great that you will soon look forward to the next time when you can sit quietly and tap your inner serenity.

The easiest way to get started is to use the TriEnergetics relaxation recording, available at our Web site (www.trienergetics.com). If you don't have the recording, don't worry. You can create your own calming environment.

There's nothing to learn, nothing for you to memorize. Just take a few minutes out of your busy schedule, sit quietly, concentrate on your breathing, and listen.

PREPARING FOR MEDITATION

Choose a quiet place where you won't be disturbed. Wear comfortable, loose-fitting clothes and loosen your belt. Most people like the lights off, or on low, but you should do whatever feels right. Some people enjoy soft scents, like lavender or sandalwood, to cleanse the air and aid relaxation. Again, that choice is up to you.

Once you find the right location, sit down. You don't have to cross your legs or sit on a cushion in the lotus position; just sit comfortably in a chair or on the floor. Keep your back straight, with your head set squarely on your shoulders. Don't lean forward or backward.

EXERCISE: The Healing Light Meditation

The Healing Light meditation is a powerful technique to help you relax.

- Begin by imagining a beam of brilliant, warm light illuminating your body. If you have trouble imagining the light, simply focus your attention on your body, concentrating on feeling sensations of warmth and comfort.

- Concentrate the light on the top of your head. Feel the warmth of this light as it gently caresses your scalp. Feel the light relaxing your scalp muscles, making them feel warm and soft. Feel the tension melt away. Feel the muscles start to tingle.

- Next, imagine the light as it slowly moves down your body. Feel it on your forehead and temples, gently warming them, relaxing them. Feel your temples begin to tingle as the warm sensation grows. Then move the light down over your cheeks, down to your jaw, feeling the warmth the whole time. Feel your jaw relax and hang open slightly. Feel the tension melt away.

- Slowly, move the light to your neck, warming and relaxing the muscles on the front and back, gently massaging them with the light's warm, healing power. Feel your neck muscles relax and loosen. Feel them grow warmer.

- Then move the light down to your shoulders, arms, hands, chest, abdomen, pelvis, thighs, knees, calves, feet, and toes. Take the time to fully relax each individual muscle. Focus your attention on the light's warmth as it melts the tension away.

- Finally, feel your entire body basking in this wonderful, warm beam of light. Feel it relax and loosen.

- Feel it warm and tingle.

You could do this same exercise imagining a warm waterfall gently flowing down your body. Whichever imagery you use, the goal is to focus your mind on the relaxation of your body.

KEYS TO MEDITATION

While there's nothing mystical about how to meditate, we'd like to offer some suggestions to help you get the most out of your meditation practice.

Keep Breathing

The way that you breathe while you meditate is extremely important. The next chapter will discuss the essential breathing techniques for relaxation, but you don't need to read that chapter in order to get started.

The important thing to know is that while relaxing your muscles, you should breathe deeply. Slowly, take a very deep breath in through your nose and allow your abdomen to bulge as you breathe. Think of the fresh air entering your body as warm, vital energy. Direct it to all parts of your body. Allow it to fill you and relax you.

As you exhale, think of the air leaving your lungs, taking your tension with it. Think *energy in, tension out.* Notice how your body relaxes as you let go. As tension leaves your body, see if you can release it even more. Every exhaled breath is an opportunity to let go.

Be aware of your breathing. Notice how you breathe in. Notice how you breathe out. Don't try to control your breath. Don't force it.

You might notice that your breathing gets slower and shallower as the meditation progresses. This happens when you become more relaxed; your body requires less oxygen because your metabolism has slowed down.

Thought Bubbles

Perhaps you enjoy the beginning of a meditation, but then you start to think about other things. As soon as these thoughts pop into your head, you try to force them out, which only makes you think more. Soon, you're bombarded with thoughts about work and home and family and unpaid bills, and you become tense again.

Don't worry about thoughts while you meditate. Don't try to force them from your mind. Thoughts will come, because your mind won't stop thinking for more than a few seconds at a time. It is the nature of the mind to think.

The phenomenon of the mind thinking is similar to champagne bubbles floating from the bottom of a glass to the surface. Champagne always bubbles. Thoughts come from the deep recesses of the mind and float to the surface. The mind always thinks.

You can't stop your mind from thinking, so what you need to do is learn how to let your thoughts go. When a thought comes, just watch it. Observe the thought, but don't engage with it. Be aware that you're thinking, but don't develop any opinions or judgments about the thought. Just let it float to the surface of your consciousness like a champagne bubble.

Then observe the next thought as it floats into your awareness. Then the next. Just let them flow.

Don't Worry, Be Happy

When you're meditating, don't worry about how you're doing. As soon as you start to wonder whether you're relaxing properly, you shift from a state of relaxation to one of anxiety. If you notice that you're either becoming absorbed in a thought or judging your progress, shift your attention back to your breath and focus on releasing tension. Imagine the warm, healing light again.

Remember, your mind will wander. This is not a problem. Just practice bringing your attention back to your breath. Observe your thoughts peacefully. When you do this, you're training your mind to become aware, and this new awareness will carry over into your daily life.

Mantras

If you like, you may choose a focus word or phrase to use while you meditate, one that evokes a special meaning for you. Many schools of meditation use such a focus word, also called a *mantra*. The purpose of a mantra is to help trigger your relaxation and act as a focus for your attention.

You can choose any word or sound that you wish. The goal is to find something that evokes pleasant sensations and helps you relax. An example of a mantra would be the word "meadow," which for most people evokes calm pictures. Search around until you find the right word for you.

If you find a word that you'd like to use, repeat it to yourself over and over in your mind. Take a deep breath and repeat the sound with each exhalation. Allow the word to take you deeper and deeper into that relaxed state.

You don't have to use a mantra. Many people focus only on their breath. It doesn't matter which you choose to do, just enjoy the process.

Ten Minutes a Day for a New You

In contrast to cardiovascular training, it's hard to say exactly how long you should sit and practice relaxation. In some ways, the more you can meditate, the better. However, a reasonable goal is to sit for a minimum of ten minutes daily.

Practice is indispensable to progress. It's important that you practice meditating at least once a day. Allow yourself the time to do this.

Remember, your only goal is to sit and relax. Sometimes, it will seem that the only thing that you're doing is chasing your mind and catching up with your thoughts. Don't be discouraged. The relaxation response is still most likely occurring in your body. Long before you think that you're meditating properly, you will notice that you feel more peaceful. More importantly, you will be reducing stress and training yourself to manage the stress in your life.

Moving On

We've just discussed how important breathing is to meditation. In the next chapter, we'll show you how good breathing can benefit every area of your life.

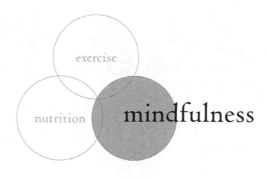

exercise

nutrition

mindfulness

chapter 9

The Breath of Life: Deep Breathing for Health and Vitality

Breathing. It seems so simple, doesn't it? Breathe in. Breathe out. Breathe in. Breathe out. You don't even have to think about it, you just do it all day long. In the car, on the job, at the mall. You even do it in your sleep. What could be simpler?

But what would you say if we told you that 95 percent of all Americans are breathing wrong?

Breathing wrong? How can I breathe wrong? you might think. *I'm still here, aren't I? I'm inhaling and exhaling; isn't that all there is to it?*

No. Believe it or not, you probably don't know how to breathe properly, and as a result, your body may be suffering. Poor breathing is one of the many important factors that can set you up for developing disease.

Disease? you ask. Yes, disease.

Poor breathing robs your body of necessary oxygen. Poor breathing triggers the catecholamine stress cascade. Poor breathing causes your muscles to tighten into knots of tension, increases your blood pressure, and increases your risk of stroke and heart attack.

And right now, as you read this book, hunched up in your chair or propped up in bed, you are probably breathing poorly. We bet that before you started reading this chapter, you weren't aware of your breath at all.

BREATHING IS POWERFUL

You're certainly not alone. Most people in this country aren't aware of their breath. They don't realize that there is more than one way to breathe. They don't know how to breathe in a way that maximizes the body's tissue concentration of oxygen and eliminates carbon dioxide most effectively. They don't know how to breathe in a way that calms the body, slows the heart, lowers the blood pressure, and decreases the production of free radicals. They don't know how to breathe in a way that helps the body eliminate stress.

Now, it may be hard to believe that something you've done every minute of your life without even thinking about it could bring so much benefit to the body if done properly and be so harmful if done improperly, so we wouldn't be surprised if your next question were *Can breathing do all that?* The answer is yes.

BAD BREATHING

Okay, but what is bad breathing?

During one of our first seminars, before we started to talk about the benefits of proper breathing, we asked each of our participants to take a deep breath. That's all—just take a deep breath.

This was a group of overly stressed professionals who were trying to improve their lives and their health. Even before coming to us, many of them had started exercise regimens, learned some of the principles of proper nutrition, and even lost weight. For the most part, they were pretty confident that they were on the right path toward living well.

But when asked to take a deep breath, invariably they all did the same things, as if following a choreographed routine. Each one looked up, sat straight, squared the shoulders, and then tried to suck as much air as possible into the chest. They all thought that to take a deep breath meant to expand the ribs, puff out the chest, and suck in that air.

That is bad breathing.

How to Breathe Wrong

1. Straighten your spine and neck.

2. Square up your shoulders.

3. Expand your chest as much as possible.

But isn't this what we all do every time we take a deep breath? When the doctor says, "Take a deep breath," we all do the same chest-expanding routine. In fact, a very popular health author described in her book the amount of chest expansion that one should have to be considered a good breather. She included detailed directions about how to use a tape measure to determine the difference in chest circumference between inhalation and exhalation.

This is wrong. Good breathing comes from the belly, not the chest.

Proper breathing is a science and an art. It is something that you must work on, consciously, every day. You don't have to meditate to breathe correctly, nor do you have to burn incense or light candles. All it takes is practice and diligence. In this chapter, we'll show you how to breathe for health and vitality. The rewards will be tremendous.

BREATH AND THE ANCIENT WAY

Breath was a central concept of Taoist philosophy more than two thousand years ago. The act of breathing was thought to bring *qi,* or life energy, into the body. Qi, the vital element in air, was considered so important that it was literally regarded as a nutrient, and an entire science, *qi gong,* or breathing exercise, developed as a formal branch of Chinese medicine.

The Taoist sages observed that when an animal, such as a puppy, took a breath, it was primarily the abdomen that expanded. Yet, when a man took a breath, most of the expansion was in the chest, with little movement of the belly. They noted how effortlessly the puppy drew each breath, while the man seemed to labor for air.

These sages realized, thousands of years ago, that breathing was the only vital function that bridged voluntary and involuntary control. They noticed that they couldn't consciously control the constriction of their blood vessels or the peristalsis of their intestines, but they could control their breath. They also realized that owing to the pivotal role breathing played between mind and body, correct breathing could regulate all other functions, including pulse, blood pressure, digestion, metabolism, and hormone secretion.

Two thousand years later, we are just beginning to discover scientifically what the sages observed empirically. They were right.

WHY BREATHING MATTERS

> Breathing is the first place, not the last, one should look when fatigue, disease, or other evidence of disordered energy presents itself.
> —Sheldon Saul Hendler

Before we get into the mechanics of proper breathing—and teach you the new choreographed routine that we want you to follow—we'd like to show you why breathing properly is so important and explain the physiologic difference between good and bad breathing. As we'll tell you over and over again, awareness of your breath is vital to your health and well-being.

Take a moment and perform this quick exercise to familiarize yourself with your breathing habits. You'll need a watch or clock with a second hand.

EXERCISE: Noticing How You Breathe

Sit in a quiet room that is well ventilated and at a comfortable temperature. Breathe as you normally do. Keep in mind that the simple act of concentrating on your breathing will alter it to some degree. When you first concentrate on your breathing, you'll tend to hold your breath or breathe slower than usual. Try not to do this. Keep your breath as natural as possible. Let it flow.

First, use a watch to count the breaths you take in thirty seconds. Multiply this by two and you have your breathing rate. What is it?

Now take a moment and simply observe your breathing.

Where is the greatest amount of body movement when you inhale? In your chest? In your shoulders and upper arms?

Does your breathing seem regular or irregular? Are your breaths deep or shallow? Do you feel satisfied after each breath?

Now, take a deep breath. A really deep breath. What do you notice? Do you feel yourself move upward when you inhale? Do you notice your head moving backward when you inhale? Do you feel restriction in your chest or solar plexus?

Put your hand on your abdomen. When you take a deep breath, do you feel your belly expand, or is most of the movement in your chest and rib cage?

Now imagine that you are in a terrible traffic jam. Your hands are gripping the steering wheel; your knuckles are turning white with frustration. Imagine your foot pounding on the brake, over and over again. You're running twenty minutes late for an important meeting, or you're late to pick up the kids. Drivers are honking behind you. You're late! A cop pulls up behind you. A truck cuts you off in front. You're late!

Can you feel this scene? Really imagine it? Notice what happens to your breathing as you visualize this scene. Do you breathe faster? More shallowly? How deep are your breaths? Where do those breaths come from? Do you feel tension gather in your chest?

Measure your breathing rate again. Has it changed? How do you feel after each breath? Satisfied? Still hungry for air? How about the rest of your body? Do you feel stress or tension?

This seems like such a simple test, but there is so much information to be gained. If you were honest in allowing your breath to come naturally, you probably noticed that your breathing came mainly from your chest and that when you took a deep breath, your rib cage expanded considerably, your shoulders squared, and your head tilted back slightly.

This is the typical posture of a chest breather.

Chest breathing is the result of years of nonawareness of the breath combined with just as many years of stress. Stress-related tension makes your body tight and tense, restricting your natural breathing motions. Chest breathing is the way most people breathe. Unfortunately, it is bad for your health.

BELLY BREATHING IS GOOD BREATHING

Belly breathing is the natural, correct way to breathe, yet so few people do it. Stress and tension rob you of your ability to perform even this most basic act. When you hold tension in your back, shoulders, and arms, these muscles are primed to contract with each breath. When you wear tight clothing and buckle your belt one notch too tight, you constrict the natural motion of the belly necessary for good breathing.

When you walk around with your belly tight and firm, sucking in your gut, you are doing everything possible to rob yourself of life-giving oxygen. But you can have a hard, flat stomach and still allow it to be loose and free for each breath. You just have to learn how. In this chapter, we'll show you how to control your stress and improve your health in the easiest, most effective way you will ever discover: by belly breathing.

Ten Wonderful Benefits of Belly Breathing

> improved sense of calm and well-being

> improved ability to handle stress

> better control over emotional upset

> lower blood pressure

> calmer heart rate

> improved digestion

> decreased muscle tension

> improved body oxygenation

> improved muscular relaxation

> improved control over panic attacks

THE MECHANICS OF BREATHING

Here's a quick anatomy lesson that will help you understand why belly breathing is so important.

THE DIAPHRAGM IS YOUR MOST POWERFUL BREATHING MUSCLE

The major muscle of respiration (breathing) is the diaphragm. You've probably heard that before. But what exactly is the diaphragm?

The *diaphragm* is a large muscle that separates your chest cavity (lungs and heart) from your abdominal cavity (stomach and intestines). Believe it or not, the diaphragm is actually the most powerful muscle in the entire body. It works constantly—all day, all night—and never fatigues.

The diaphragm is attached all along the circumference of the lower chest cavity. Think of it as a trampoline separating your chest from your belly. In its relaxed position, the diaphragm curves upward in a dome shape.

Now, when you take a deep breath, the diaphragm contracts; the trampoline gets pulled tight. The diaphragm pulls down toward the abdomen, flattening from its dome shape. This creates a vacuum in the lungs and sucks in air.

What else happens? Since the diaphragm separates the chest from the belly, when the diaphragm contracts, it enlarges the chest cavity and decreases the space in the abdomen. The downward movement of the diaphragm displaces the intestines, causing the belly to bulge outward.

When you exhale, the diaphragm relaxes to its natural position, the belly returns to its normal state, and the air is expelled from the lungs.

Breathe in from the diaphragm, belly expands. Breathe out from the diaphragm, belly returns.

CHEST BREATHING IMMOBILIZES THE DIAPHRAGM

When you breathe from your chest, holding your belly tight, you paralyze the diaphragm. You incapacitate the main breathing muscle of your body.

When you do this, you force the chest muscles (the *intercostals*) and a few other small muscles to do all the work. These puny muscles are much weaker than the diaphragm and are only designed to be accessory muscles of respiration. They are meant to be used only when breathing is greatly increased, like during exertion or illness. They simply cannot expand the lungs to their fullest capacity. They don't have the power.

But don't believe us; find out for yourself.

EXERCISE: Chest Breathing vs. Diaphragm Breathing

Take a deep chest breath. Hold your belly tight, as tight as you can, and inhale deeply from your chest. Expand it to the max. Suck in as much air as you can. Keep that belly tight! Be aware of how long you can inhale comfortably and how much air enters your lungs.

Now allow your belly to relax—really relax. Take a deep breath from the belly. Expand your belly with the breath, pooch it out, allow the breath to sink low into your abdomen. Breathe in as much air as you can.

What difference do you notice? With the belly breath, you should be able to inhale much longer, bringing more air into your lungs. You also may notice that the belly breath is somewhat more satisfying, satiating your need for oxygen and requiring less energy. Belly breathing is more comfortable than chest breathing.

The intercostals simply are not designed to be your primary breathing muscles.

● Todd's Tale: Don't Be a Pink Puffer

When I was an intern working in the hospital, I took care of a tremendous number of patients with emphysema. These patients, suffering from terrible lung disease due to years of smoking, were called "pink puffers" by other doctors because they puffed and puffed but could never get enough oxygen into their lungs. Watching their breathing, I could see their intercostals pumping away, trying to get air into their diseased lungs. The effort was not very successful. Unfortunately, it was too late for these patients to learn belly breathing, because their lungs were too badly damaged to breathe effectively. But it's not too late for you. If you continue to breathe from your chest, you ignore your primary muscle of respiration and deprive yourself of life-giving oxygen. Don't let that happen!

CHEST BREATHING IS INEFFICIENT

Let's continue with the anatomy lesson. The *air sacs* are the vital structures in the lungs that absorb oxygen into the bloodstream and also eliminate the carbon dioxide that your body has produced. To reach the air sacs, the air must pass through the *trachea* (windpipe) and the two main *bronchial tubes.*

But here's the problem: the trachea and bronchial tubes don't have air sacs. They are only big tubes. This means that all the air that is inside these major passageways is useless to the body. It's like traffic stuck in the Lincoln Tunnel. It doesn't do anything. It doesn't provide oxygen or release carbon dioxide. The trachea and bronchial tubes are dead space.

The average person has about 150 cubic centimeters of dead space inside the lungs. That's about the volume of a soda can.

The amount of air you inhale and exhale during an unconscious breath is your *tidal volume.* For an average person, this is about 400 to 500 cubic centimeters of air.

Now think about that for a minute. With a typical breath, you inhale only 400 cubic centimeters of air—air that is supposed to supply the brain and the body with all the oxygen needed to function properly. But 150 cubic centimeters of that air is stuck in dead space. Only 250 cubic centimeters of air is getting into the lungs with each breath.

A typical chest breath brings into the lungs only a fraction of what's possible. And a lot of the air that is brought in is dead air. Worthless air. This is horribly inefficient breathing.

BELLY BREATHING IS EFFICIENT

When you breathe with your diaphragm, with your belly, you can greatly increase the total amount of air breathed into your lungs, increase the amount of air driven into the air sacs, exchange more oxygen, release more carbon dioxide, and better overcome the dead space. These are scientific facts.

Good belly breathers can double or even triple their tidal volume in only a few days of practice. Belly breathers can bring in more than a liter (that's 1,000 cubic centimeters) of air with each breath. When you belly breathe, your respiration rate drops, you work less, and you get more oxygen to your body.

Breathing from the belly is better breathing.

GO WITH THE FLOW

The purpose of breathing is, of course, to get oxygen into the body and to release carbon dioxide. Carbon dioxide is a waste product of the body's normal, healthy metabolism. It must be excreted properly, or else it can cause some serious health problems.

In order for the body to do all of this, the heart pumps blood to the lungs. The air sacs absorb oxygen and transport it to the bloodstream, while they simultaneously take the carbon dioxide from the blood and release it into the lungs so it can be exhaled.

As you now know, when you breathe with your chest, you bring in only a small fraction of the air that your lungs could hold. This tiny amount of air expands the tops of the lungs (the area in your upper chest), but there isn't enough air to expand the lower, deeper portions of the lungs. Those portions remain unused, collapsed.

But did you know that less than one-tenth of a liter of blood flows through the top of the lungs every minute, while over a liter flows through the bottom portion during that same minute?

Think about that. With each shallow chest breath, most of the blood flow to the lungs is going to the lower portions, which aren't even getting air. All that blood is wasted. Only a fraction of your total blood flow is being oxygenated with each breath.

Each of those shallow breaths is robbing you of the precious oxygen that you need to live. This means that in your body there could be a severe shortage of available oxygen and a dangerous buildup of carbon dioxide.

In order to get enough oxygen into your blood, your heart has to pump faster and harder to get more blood flowing through the tops of the lungs. You also have to breathe harder and faster to take in enough air to oxygenate that blood. This places stress on your heart and triggers the catecholamine cascade.

Bad breathing creates internal stress that you can feel and guides you down the pathway toward heart disease.

Deep belly breathing, on the other hand, opens up those lower, deeper portions of the lungs. It oxygenates your blood effectively and removes harmful carbon dioxide. This actually allows your heart to slow down and relax. In turn, this has an amazing calming effect on the body as it turns off your stress-induced catecholamine cascade.

BELLY BREATHING IMPROVES DIGESTION

There's one more advantage to belly breathing over chest breathing. With each deep inhalation, as the diaphragm contracts, it massages the organs of the abdomen. This massaging action actually improves blood flow to the intestines and the stomach, facilitates the movement of food through your intestines, and improves your digestion. This can help to eliminate problems such as constipation, diarrhea, and belly pain.

All that from breathing properly!

> ### Six Physiologic Benefits of Belly Breathing
> › Expands lung capacity
> › Maximizes contribution from the diaphragm
> › Maximizes oxygen intake to overcome dead space
> › Expands lower portions of the lungs to maximize circulation-to-oxygen ratio
> › Maximizes oxygen–carbon dioxide gas exchange
> › Enhances peristalsis of the intestines

THE ART OF BREATHING

We hope that you're now convinced that you need to change the way you draw your breath. The next question becomes, how do you learn to belly breathe?

Fortunately, the Taoist sages studied breathing in great detail, and from their teachings we have learned a lot about how to breathe properly. The Lying Belly Breath is a simple, quick exercise that you can do every day to help retrain your body to breathe in the proper, healthful way.

EXERCISE: The Lying Belly Breath

Find a private moment and a quiet room where you will not be disturbed. Lie on your back with your arms comfortably at your sides and your legs straight. Sometimes it helps to use an object such as a book as a visual aid. Place the book on your belly, just above your belly button.

Slowly inhale through your nose, with your tongue comfortably resting against the roof of your mouth. Concentrate on breathing deeply from the belly; sink the breath down as low as you can. Expand your belly as much as possible with each breath. Watch the book rise with each breath.

Slow down your breath. Take a full four or five seconds for each inhalation. Hold it for a moment, then slowly let it out, exhaling gently through your mouth. Watch the book slowly settle as you exhale. Again, let the exhalation be slow, over four or five seconds.

Breathe in through your nose; book rises. Breathe out through your mouth; book settles back down.

Repeat this calming exercise for several minutes every day.

The Lying Belly Breath is very relaxing and calming, as well as a great way to learn deep belly breathing.

Belly breathing can, of course, be practiced in any position, at any time of day.

BELLY BREATHING IN THE WORKPLACE

Practice your belly breathing while seated at your desk. Pull your chair back for a moment, take your focus off your computer screen or your work pile, and relax your body. If you're wearing pants, you may want to loosen your belt. Concentrate on a slow, gentle inhalation, sinking the breath deep in the belly. Feel the belly bulge as the diaphragm lowers into the abdomen. Again, draw out your inhalation for a full four or five seconds. Your tongue should be gently resting against the roof of your mouth.

Hold the breath briefly, then exhale. Draw out your exhalation for four or five seconds. Inhale through your nose, exhale through your mouth. Inhale. Exhale.

You can do this many times a day. Any time you feel stressed or anxious, at work or at home, allow yourself to stop for a moment. Close your eyes and concentrate on a few deep, cleansing belly breaths. You will immediately feel your tension, anger, or anxiety lessen and dissipate. Practice many times a day—between clients, between meetings, or just for a refreshing, energizing break.

BEATING THE TRAFFIC JAM

Our favorite place to concentrate on belly breathing is when we're driving. Unlike meditation, breathing can be practiced anytime, anywhere. You can practice when there's bad traffic ahead, to keep calm, or even if the road is open, just to keep yourself focused and healthy.

Turn off the radio or play a soft, pleasing tape. Avoid loud or fast music, since it will increase your heart rate, your breathing rate, and your stress level.

With both hands on the wheel and your eyes focused on the road and the traffic ahead of you, slow down your breathing. Inhale deeply through the nose, sinking the breath into the belly. Feel your belly expand. Feel the fullness. Hold it, then exhale slowly through your mouth.

The next time someone cuts you off on the freeway, try belly breathing rather than honking your horn.

BREATHING AND EMOTIONS

The way you draw your breath has a profound effect on your moment-by-moment feelings of emotional well-being. Deep belly breathing yields a calming, relaxing, pleasant sensation that allows you to concentrate on the moment. On the other hand, most of your unpleasant emotions are tied in to changes in your breathing patterns.

When you are angry, your breathing becomes tight, with an accentuated inhale and a sharp exhale. When you are sad, the pattern is reversed, with a shallow inhale and fitful, sobbing exhales. These breathing patterns can contribute to your feelings of emotional upset.

Proper breathing will not change the instigating circumstances that triggered your anger or sadness, but it can greatly alter the way you respond. Proper breathing can help you deal with negative emotions in a positive way by giving you more control over your body's response.

Try this simple exercise to explore the powerful connection between your breathing and your emotions.

EXERCISE: Using Breathing to Release Anger

Find a quiet place where you won't be disturbed. Loosen your belt or tight clothing. Sit comfortably in a chair, back straight, head and neck straight. Take a few deep, cleansing breaths.

Now imagine a scene that makes you angry—really angry. Imagine whatever it takes to get yourself worked up. Your kids, your spouse, your boss, traffic, an injustice, whatever pushes your anger button. Keep imagining that scene until you feel that anger swelling inside you, burning deep in your solar plexus. Your body becomes tight, your breathing gets shallower, your nostrils flare, your eyes burn with intensity. Really feel it!

Now take a moment and concentrate all of your energy on your breathing. Breathe deeply, from the belly. Slow down that inhalation; feel the belly expand. With a nice slow exhalation, feel the belly return. Breathe deeply from the belly for four or five breaths.

What do you notice? Most people will feel acutely aware that their anger has dissipated. The tightness in the solar plexus has relaxed, the shoulders have loosened, the body feels better.

BREATHING AND ANGER

We will venture to say that it is impossible to maintain a harsh negative emotion like anger when you exercise proper breathing. The very act of concentrating on your breath draws your focus away from the instigating stimulus and into your belly. There, while you continue to concentrate on breathing, you correct the imbalance that the anger has caused, and the body returns to a more relaxed state. The anger fades, the body heals.

Try this exercise several times until you feel this amazing change. Practice the exercise until you can consciously choose to exercise your mind's innate ability to control your body's reaction to anger or other negative emotions. Then, the next time you feel your anger rising, simply concentrate on your breath and allow that anger to pass.

BREATHING AND STRESS

As you have already gathered from chapter 8 and from this chapter, proper breathing is essential for stress management. The ancient Taoists emphasized this. They suggested using the breath as a way to nurture mindfulness, to focus on the rhythmic movement of breathing, to calm the mind, quiet the thoughts, and still worry.

Studies with biofeedback and deep-breathing techniques have demonstrated conclusively that good breath control can slow the heart, lower the blood pressure, and change the *galvanic skin response* (the way the skin conducts electricity), indicating the dissipation of stress.

BREATHING AND ANXIETY

On the other hand, improper breathing leads not only to stress and its related problems, but to anxiety and panic attacks as well. Panic attacks are not fun. You breathe and breathe but can never seem to get enough air.

● Jessica's Amazing Turnaround

We saw firsthand the connection between breathing and panic attacks when Jessica enrolled in our workshop. Her husband had died tragically not long before. One day, while getting onto the freeway, Jessica started hyperventilating, and she experienced a sudden, overwhelming fear of driving. She told us she nearly lost control of her car because her hands were shaking so badly, sweat was pouring into her eyes, her heart was pounding, and she was panting like a dog. She thought she was going to die. Finally, she had to pull to the side of the freeway and call for help.

After that, the same panic reaction occurred every time she tried to drive on the freeway. She was unable to commute to work, visit friends, or even go shopping without the twinges of panic. Her life was in shambles.

In our first workshop with her, we discussed the basics of belly breathing and guided her through a deep-breathing meditation. The very next week, she marched into the classroom and proudly yelled out that she was cured. She had been driving with no problems, even on the freeway. Whenever she felt her panic starting, she just took control of her breathing, focused on her belly, and allowed the fear to pass.

This change, she felt, was miraculous.

As much as we would like to take credit for miracles, we can't. What Jessica had learned to do was to slow down her breath, balance the level of gasses in her blood, shut off her stress cascade, and turn off the panic cycle before it started. These are learned benefits of proper breathing—the same benefits that await you.

How Overbreathing Triggers Panic Attacks

Let's take a look at the fundamental body mechanisms through which improper breathing leads to anxiety and panic attacks.

Since it is so important for the brain to receive an oxygen-rich blood supply, the arteries in the brain are very sensitive to the amounts of gasses carried in the blood. Special receptors called *carboreceptors* detect the amount of carbon dioxide in the bloodstream.

Improper breathing leads a person to breathe faster and faster. This state is called *hyperventilation* or *overbreathing*. As the breathing rate increases, more and more carbon dioxide gets blown out by the lungs, and the level of carbon dioxide in the blood drops. A single sharp exhalation can reduce your carbon dioxide level by as much as 20 percent, and breathing hard thirty times in a minute will cut your carbon dioxide level in half.

Now, reduced levels of carbon dioxide in the blood do several things. First, the arteries of the brain constrict rapidly, reducing the blood flow to the brain and causing a shortage of oxygen. Secondly, carbon dioxide is critical for the very delicate balance of acids and bases in the bloodstream. When the carbon dioxide level falls, the blood becomes too alkaline, and a condition called *respiratory alkalosis* results.

Respiratory alkalosis triggers the release of catecholamines, which causes faster and faster breathing, a pounding heart rate, shaking, and sweating. Yet all this breathing still doesn't satisfy the person, who by now is hungering for air. This faster breathing blows off even more carbon dioxide, leading to more alkalosis. This vicious circle eventually creates a full-on panic attack.

Anxiety, which plagues millions of Americans in our high-pressure, high-stress society, is in actuality a breathing disorder. That's right. The drug companies have been making a fortune peddling drugs to keep people calm, when in reality all they need to do is learn how to breathe.

Exhale the Panic

The solution, as Jessica found, is to consciously break the cycle. Concentrate your breath deep in the belly. Slow down your breathing. You can control panic, phobias, and anxiety by taking control of your breath.

It will take concentrated practice to break out of bad breathing habits. Muscle tension accumulated over a lifetime doesn't dissipate overnight. It can take up to six months to learn healthier breathing patterns and another six months before those new patterns feel as if they are second nature. But if you work at it, you will see results. Anxiety, phobias, and panic will lessen. You will feel calmer, more stable, and more relaxed.

Five TriEnergetics Tips for Better Breathing

› Don't wear constrictive clothing around the waist. The belly needs room to expand and contract.

› Watch your posture. Keep your back straight, your shoulders square, and your head lightly positioned on the top of your neck. Hunching your shoulders, bending your spine, and tilting your head forward will all restrict your airways and make breathing more difficult.

› Breathe in gently through your nose, with your tongue resting against the palate.

› Breathe from the belly, not the chest.

› When stress arises, concentrate your focus on your belly and breathe deeply. Inhale to a count of four, hold briefly, then exhale to a count of four. This will harmonize your breathing and prepare you for any stressful situation.

Moving On

The ancient Taoist sages recognized that breathing was the key to the mind-body interaction. Now this knowledge is available to you. You can control your breath, and thereby you can control your body. You can control your stress. You can control your health.

So breathe deeply.

PART 2

The TriEnergetics
Program

chapter 10

Getting Started on the TriEnergetics Program

We want you to get started on the program as quickly as possible. There is no better time to make a change than right now.

WHAT YOU'LL NEED

To get started, you will need only a few basic items.

- Comfortable workout clothes that allow for a full range of movement. No tight belts or collars!

- A pair of good walking shoes, available at any specialty sporting shoe store.

- A watch with a second hand, or a stopwatch, for timing your walk.

- A set of elastic exercise bands, available through www.trienergetics.com or at most sporting goods stores. (The elastic bands are not used until the fourth week of the program, so there is no reason to delay starting until you get these.)

- A ball the size of a soccer ball.

INTEGRATED LIVING

The goal of this program is to help you live a healthy life, fully integrating the three major energies of your health. In each weekly session of the TriEnergetics plan, you will find a new goal in each of the three major categories: body energy, mind energy, and nourishment energy. Each of these guidelines is progressive, building upon the changes you've made the week before. Best of all, each weekly recommendation is gentle and easy, never requiring you to make a huge lifestyle change all at once.

BODY ENERGY

In the body energy sections, you will find new goals in aerobic and strength-training exercise. Each week you will improve your aerobic conditioning and add another strength-building exercise to your weekly regimen. The goal is to increase your aerobic capacity, tone your muscles, build your bone strength, and firm up your body.

In addition, each week we'll give you a new Taoist stretch to help limber your body, improve your flexibility, loosen your joints, help you relax, and ward off muscle pain.

MIND ENERGY

In the mind energy sections, you will find weekly assignments in meditation, deep breathing techniques, and stress reduction strategies. The goal here is to help you combat the deleterious effects of stress on your body, while helping you to integrate your mind with the wonderful changes that are happening in your body as you proceed through the program.

NOURISHMENT ENERGY

In each nourishment energy section, you will find your weekly assignment for a slight modification in your diet. Each change has been carefully thought out by our staff of nutritionists and dietitians to give you maximum benefit with minimal effort. The goal is to move you gradually toward a healthier diet to maximize your energy, strengthen your immune system, and minimize your risk of illnesses such as heart disease.

BODY, MIND, AND NOURISHMENT WORK TOGETHER

You must make a commitment to enhance all three of the major energies of your life simultaneously for this program to work to its maximum potential. If you follow only the exercise plan or only the stress reduction plan, you will still see some pleasant changes in your body, your mood, and your energy level, but you won't get the maximal benefit unless you do all the parts at the same time.

In your body, each of these energies is connected to the others. Your nourishment will have a tremendous impact on your mood, your ability to handle stress, and your energy level. Exercise will brighten your mood, but it works best when the body's muscles are properly fueled. And simply exercising and eating well isn't enough to help you combat the overwhelming stress of daily life.

Your body is a very delicate machine. For it to run as smoothly and efficiently as possible, you must balance all three energies.

THE TRIENERGETICS WEEKLY ACTION PLAN

Each week, in addition to new goals about body, mind, and nourishment energy, we'll present you with a weekly action plan, a carefully constructed motivational exercise for you to use to maximize your commitment to the program.

We encourage you to use the action plan each week. Take the time to think about the questions and write out your answers. We've included plenty of space for you to write right in the book. There is a huge mental difference between simply thinking about the questions and actually writing out your answers. Writing will strengthen your resolve and create new pathways in your brain, committing you to improving your health. Don't miss out on this opportunity to maximize the benefits of the program.

PRETESTING

To help you get started, we've included a number of pretest forms at the end of this chapter. We've left ample space for you to fill out these forms right in the book. These worksheets will help you clarify your current health status and your needs. Once you have a clear idea of your current level of wellness, you can better focus on the changes you want to make over the next six weeks.

AN ACTIVE, HEALTHY LIFESTYLE: PLANNING YOUR WEEK

We hope you'll commit to a healthy, active TriEnergetics lifestyle seven days a week while you are working the program. It's important to pay attention to each of the body's energies on a regular basis. We encourage you to

- walk four times a week

- perform the strength-building exercises three times a week

- complete the stretches every day

- practice meditation and deep breathing every day

- practice mindful eating at least once a week

- rest on the days you don't exercise

A weekly format, then, could look like this:

	Sun	Mon	Tues	Wed	Thurs	Fri	Sat
Walking	X		X		X		X
Strength training	X		X		X		
Rest		X		X		X	
Stretching	Every morning						
Meditation/ deep breathing	Every day						
Mindful eating	Once a week						

Of course, this is only one suggestion. Any way that you make the time to fit the program into your schedule will be the best for you. Your schedule should be flexible enough that if you miss a day of walking or strength training, you can simply pick it up again the next day.

GETTING STARTED

Here are the preliminary steps to take in body energy, mind energy, nourishment energy, mindful eating, and supplementation.

BODY ENERGY

To get started on the exercise program, we want you to perform a timed one-mile walk. Use your car to measure out a one-mile walking course near your home or work. You can walk over any terrain you choose, whether in a park, along the seashore, or simply around the block. Once you've measured your course, you'll need to make sure that you have a proper pair of walking shoes and comfortable clothes.

Start your stopwatch and begin walking your course. Don't run, and don't walk too quickly. This isn't a race. The goal is simply to see how quickly you can comfortably walk one mile. A good pace would be one that is

159

slightly beyond conversational, meaning that you could carry on a conversation while you walked, but it would take some effort.

Once you've finished your mile, stop the watch and allow yourself to cool down by breathing deeply.

Record the time it took you to walk this mile here and on the Week One Pretesting form. This will be an important number for your future walking exercises.

My Timed One-Mile Walk

Date: _____

Time: _____

MIND ENERGY

We'd like you to get started on the meditation routine the very first day. Everyone who has enrolled in our seminars has taken to this routine with enthusiasm. We bet that you, like our seminar participants, have a need for some peaceful, quiet time in your hectic life. In chapter 8, we discuss the benefits of a regular meditation practice and provide a basic meditation exercise to get you started.

To get the most benefit from meditation, make a time for yourself when you can sit undisturbed. If you have the TriEnergetics meditation recording, you can use it each day to help you along. If not, simply concentrate on breathing deeply into your belly and allow your body to relax.

Once you have experienced the tranquility of deep relaxation, you will find yourself looking forward to the next time that you can sit peacefully.

NOURISHMENT ENERGY

The TriEnergetics nourishment program is carefully planned to help you gradually modify your eating habits. It's easy to do. The changes may seem small, but remember, they are cumulative. What you do the first week carries over to the second week, and the first and second weeks' changes carry over to the third week, and so on. By the time you have completed the six-week program, you will have made significant changes in your eating habits.

INTEGRATING YOUR MIND AND YOUR EATING

In chapter 5, we introduced you to the concept of mindful eating. By practicing mindful eating, you'll find eating to be a relaxing, calming experience. You'll enjoy your food more, and you will learn to recognize just how much food your body actually needs. You'll learn to stop eating when you are no longer hungry instead of continuing to eat until you are stuffed. Mindful eating is also a wonderful meditative practice.

We don't expect you to eat mindfully all of the time, only occasionally. Once a week would be an ideal way to start the practice. When you practice the exercise, concentrate on it. Make it pleasurable and relaxing.

Once you learn to stop overeating, you'll be amazed at how easily the excess weight comes off.

ANTIOXIDANT SUPPLEMENTS

Begin taking the supplements the first week. As you learned in chapter 6, your body is at war with free radicals, unseen enemies that are aging you and damaging your cells. Protect yourself by building up your defenses with antioxidants, vitamins, and minerals.

Moving On

Now you should be ready to get started. Before you do, consult with your physician if you have diabetes, high blood pressure, or elevated cholesterol; if you've had an abnormal cardiogram; or if you are a heavy smoker. In fact, if you have any question about your health, we suggest that you get your doctor's approval before you begin the program.

We want you to succeed. We're here to support you in any way that we can. If any questions come up, contact us through our Web site at www.trienergetics.com and we'll get back to you as soon as possible.

Enjoy the program; enjoy the results!

Date: _____

PHYSICAL ACTIVITY HISTORY

What type of activities do you do regularly and how much time each week do you spend doing them? Examples include walking, dancing, golf, tennis, biking, aerobics, and swimming.

Activity	Times per Week	Minutes per Activity
_____	_____	_____
_____	_____	_____
_____	_____	_____
_____	_____	_____
_____	_____	_____
_____	_____	_____

Do you like to do these activities alone or with others? _____

Do you perform other physical activities of daily living, such as housework, gardening, or climbing stairs? If yes, list type and amount.

_____

_____

Are you interested in becoming more active? ☐ Yes, right now
  ☐ Yes, but I can't right now   ☐ No, but I will think it over
  ☐ No, not now   ☐ No, I'm not interested

If yes, what types of physical activity could you see yourself doing regularly?

_____

_____

If no, why not?

_____

_____

Date: _____

DO YOU WANT TO CHANGE YOUR LIFESTYLE?

Have you made any changes in your lifestyle that you feel good about?

☐ Yes   ☐ No

If yes, what changes have you made? _____
_____

If changes could be made in your lifestyle to improve your health (for example, eating or exercise), would you be open to the changes?

☐ Yes   ☐ No

If yes, who will support and encourage you as you make these changes?

_____
_____

If no, what would keep you from making these changes?

_____
_____

What changes would you like to make?

☐ Improve my eating habits

☐ Improve my activity level

☐ Lower my blood pressure

☐ Improve my cholesterol level

☐ Get more information

☐ Learn how to prevent high or low blood glucose levels

☐ Feel better about my health

☐ Learn how to manage my weight

☐ Improve my energy level

☐ Control food cravings

☐ Improve my blood glucose control

☐ Other _____
_____
_____

Date: _____

NUTRITION HISTORY

Have you ever wanted to make changes in what you eat?   ☐ Yes   ☐ No

    If yes, what advice have you been given? _____

    _____

Are you following any type of meal plan (such as exchange lists, calorie counting, or carbohydrate counting), or restricted diet (low cholesterol, low fat, or low sodium)?

    ☐ Yes   ☐ No

    If yes, please describe _____

If yes, how much of the time are you able to follow your meal plan?

    ☐ Rarely   ☐ Sometimes   ☐ Often   ☐ Usually

How many people live in your household? _____ What ages? _____

Who usually does the cooking? _____ The shopping? _____

How many times each week do you eat away from home? _____

    Which meals are usually eaten away from home? _____

    In which type of restaurant do you eat or carry out?
    (mark F for frequently, O for occasionally, N for never)

    Fast food (hamburger, chicken, seafood, pizza, subs, tacos) _____

    Buffets/all-you-can-eat _____ Sweets/dessert shops _____

    Sit-down Restaurants _____ types: _____

Do you drink alcohol?   ☐ Beer   ☐ Wine   ☐ Liquor

    How often? _____ How much? _____

Do you take vitamins, minerals, herbs, or any other food or nutritional supplement?

    ☐ Yes   ☐ No   If yes, please list _____

Do you regularly skip meals?   ☐ Yes   ☐ No

    If yes, which meals and why? _____

Do you have "trigger" foods that often cause you to overeat?

☐ Yes   ☐ No

If yes, please list _____

Have you ever been on an extreme diet (such as fasting) or a fad diet?

☐ Yes   ☐ No

If yes, please describe _____

Do you eat for reasons other than hunger?   ☐ Yes   ☐ No

If yes, please describe _____

_____

Date: _____

WEIGHT HISTORY

Height _____ Present Weight _____ Usual Weight _____

Has your weight changed any over the past year?　☐ Yes　☐ No

    If yes, please describe how _____

_____

    How do you feel about your weight right now? _____

_____

What has been your weight range as an adult? _____

What would you consider a healthy weight for you? _____

Would you feel comfortable at that weight?　☐ Yes　☐ No

Have you ever tried to change your weight before?　☐ Yes　☐ No

    If yes, what have you tried? _____

_____

    Have you been successful? _____

_____

Are you interested in working to change your weight?

    ☐ Yes, right now

    ☐ Yes, but I can't right now

    ☐ No, not now

    ☐ No, I'm not interested

Date: _____

PHYSICAL ACTIVITY READINESS QUESTIONNAIRE (PAR-Q)

The completion of PAR-Q is a sensible first step to take if you are planning to increase the amount of physical activity in your life. For most people, physical activity should not pose any problem or hazard. PAR-Q has been designed to identify the small number of adults for whom physical activity might be inappropriate or those who should have medical advice concerning the type of activity most suitable for them.

    Common sense is your best guide in answering these questions. Please read them carefully and check the correct answer next to each question.

	Yes	No
1. Has your doctor ever said you have heart trouble?	☐	☐
2. Do you frequently have pains in your heart or chest?	☐	☐
3. Do you often feel faint or have spells of severe dizziness?	☐	☐
4. Has your doctor ever said your blood pressure was too high?	☐	☐
5. Has your doctor told you that you have a bone or joint problem such as arthritis that has been aggravated by exercise or might be made worse with exercise?	☐	☐
6. Is there a good physical reason not mentioned here why you should not follow an activity program even if you wanted to?	☐	☐
7. Are you over age sixty-five and not accustomed to vigorous exercise?	☐	☐

IF YOU ANSWERED YES TO ONE OR MORE QUESTIONS

* If you have not recently done so, consult with your personal physician by telephone or in person before increasing your physical activity or taking a fitness appraisal, such as the timed one-mile walk. Tell your doctor which questions you answered yes to on the PAR-Q or present your copy of PAR-Q.
* After medical evaluation, seek advice from your physician as to your suitability for unrestricted physical activity that starts off easily and progresses gradually.

IF YOU ANSWERED NO TO ALL QUESTIONS

* If you answered the PAR-Q questions accurately, you have reasonable assurance of your present suitability for a graduated exercise program.

WEEK ONE PRETESTING

Date: _____

INSTRUCTIONS

Resting Heart Rate

Supplies needed: stopwatch or watch with second hand

While seated, position your fingertips on your carotid artery (the large artery in your neck). This is located at the side of the Adam's apple, just below your jawbone. Press firmly but lightly to feel your pulse. Count the number of beats for fifteen seconds and multiply by four for your beats per minute. Record at the end of this worksheet.

Blood Pressure and Blood Cholesterol

To be taken at a location of your choice. Some pharmacies provide this service.

Weight and Measurements

We suggest you have another person measure you. If no one is available, you can do it yourself. Stand erect with good posture. The person measuring should pull the tape firmly but not too tightly, applying even pressure without compressing the underlying tissue. Round numbers off to the nearest quarter inch and record at the bottom of this worksheet.

Arms: At midbicep.

Chest: At the nipple line and at the midpoint of a normal breath.

Waist: At the narrowest part of the torso, below the rib cage and just above the top of the hip bone.

Hips: At the widest part.

Thighs: With legs slightly apart, at the maximum circumference, just below the gluteal fold.

One-Mile Power Walk

Supplies needed: stopwatch, flat surface, good walking shoes, writing paper and pen

After you have marked off a one-mile flat course, take a short warm-up. Then start the stopwatch and begin the one-mile walk. The purpose of this test is to see how fast you can comfortably walk a mile and to measure your ending heart rate. Try to keep a steady pace throughout. Walk, don't run. If it seems easy, walk faster. At the end of the mile, record your time and take your heart rate. Hint: Carry a scratch pad and pen to record your results. You can transfer the numbers to this worksheet later.

PRETESTING DATA

Resting heart rate _____ Blood pressure _____

Blood cholesterol _____ Weight _____

Measurements: Arms _____ Chest _____ Waist _____

               Hips _____ Thighs _____

Timed one-mile walk _____ Heart rate after one-mile walk _____

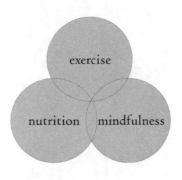

chapter 11

Week One

The longest journey begins with a single step.

—ancient proverb

We're going to be your companions on a trip that you may have been putting off for a long time: a trip to better health and to a new you. Along the way, there will be occasional stops to learn some new facts to better understand the direction you're taking. None of the steps are difficult, and you can set your own pace.

So let's get started. Relax and enjoy the program. Looking better and feeling younger is a serious goal, but that doesn't mean you can't enjoy the process of attaining it.

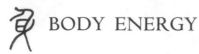

BODY ENERGY

WALKING

The first week, we're going to ease you into the program. We chose walking as the basic cardiovascular activity for the program because it offers so much, especially when you are beginning.

- Walking doesn't require special equipment or special skills.

- It is a pleasurable activity that exercises your heart, your lungs, and some of the major muscle groups of your body.

- You burn calories when you walk, about 100 calories per mile, so by walking you can lose weight.

- Walking gives you an opportunity to practice the abdominal breathing program.

To get started, you'll need to finish your pretest forms and perform the timed one-mile walk. Once you've completed your timed walk, schedule yourself enough time to walk a mile at that pace four times a week. Allow a little extra time so that you can really enjoy yourself. Give yourself a chance to savor the walk. Look at the walking exercise as your special time, a time to give yourself a treat.

Five Great Reasons to Walk for Your Health

➤ You'll live longer.

➤ You'll burn more calories.

➤ You'll lose weight.

➤ You'll build stronger bones.

➤ You'll sleep better.

This week the goal is simply to match the pace you set for yourself with your timed one-mile pretest walk. Use your stopwatch to time each walk, with the goal of meeting that pace each time.

While you are walking, pay attention to your breath. Focus on moving the air in and out with your belly, not by expanding and contracting your chest. When you do deep abdominal breathing, not only will you be improving the oxygen flow to your body, but you will also be doing a form of meditation. This will change your focus away from the stress in your life, away from your cares and woes, to the sensations of just being in your body.

Use your walk as a time to get in touch with your body. Feel the changes you make as you move your legs and your arms. Experiment with taking long strides and notice how the resultant stretching feels to your calves and to the muscles that extend your legs.

Get into the walk mentally and enjoy being in your body. You will be amazed at how quickly a mile goes by.

How fast should you walk? Remember, you are walking a timed mile. Aim for the time you recorded when you walked your pretest mile. Walk fast enough that you feel like you are exerting yourself a little, but not so fast that you become short of breath or unable to talk.

What if you are not able to comfortably walk a mile? Stay within your limitations and only gradually increase your distance.

What if you want to walk more than a mile or if you want to walk more than four days a week? No problem. You can do more if you want to, but it is not necessary for the program. You will make great progress staying within the guidelines.

STRETCHING

Stretching should be a part of your daily routine. Most people realize that stretching is essential to warm up the body and prevent injury before exercising, but stretching should not be relegated to a habitual preexercise activity. The benefits of stretching as a daily routine are far ranging and can have a dramatic impact on your sense of well-being.

When you were a baby, you had a very supple body. But as you grew older, you developed habitual patterns of muscle tension and contraction in response to pain, emotional upset, and stress. As the years pass, this can lead to a stiffer, more rigid body and headaches, backaches, and chronic pain. What you need to do is loosen up and re-create your once young, supple body.

Health Benefits of a Regular Stretching Routine

> Reduces muscle tension and makes the body feel more relaxed.

> Helps coordination by allowing for freer and easier movement.

> Calms the mind when performed as meditation.

> Increases range of motion.

> Prevents injuries such as muscle strains.

> Makes strenuous activities easier.

> Develops body awareness. As you stretch various parts of the body, you focus on them and get in touch with them. You get to know yourself.

> Helps loosen the mind's control of the body, relaxing years of emotional, physical, and psychological pain stored in the muscles.

> Promotes circulation.

> Promotes well-being.

A great time to stretch is early in the morning, when you're stiff from lying in bed all night. We recommend that you make it part of your daily routine to rise from a peaceful night's sleep and stretch to start your day.

You don't have to limit stretching to the mornings, however. Stretching is an excellent stress relieving technique. Anytime during the day or evening, particularly if you're feeling anxious or your body feels tight, take a few moments to perform your stretching routine. You'll find it can make an amazing improvement in your mood, your stress level, and the way your body feels.

The first stretch we'd like you to begin doing is the Great Tai-Chi Circle Breath.

EXERCISE: The Great Tai-Chi Circle Breath

This highly fluid exercise synchronizes the body, breath, and mind. It is one of the best breathing exercises in the entire Taoist repertoire.

Posture

- Stand with your heels together, toes angled out at forty-five degrees.

- Keep your knees slightly bent, your spine erect.

- Bring your hands together in front, below the navel, palms up, with your right hand cupped in your left (fig. 11.1).

Technique

1. Empty your lungs thoroughly and commence a long, slow inhalation through the nostrils. As you inhale, slowly raise your hands out to the sides, palms up (fig. 11.2).

2. Bring both hands up above your head, palms up, in one slow, fluid movement, inscribing as wide a circle as possible. At the same time, slowly straighten your knees and continue inhaling until your lungs are full (fig. 11.3).

3. Begin a slow, controlled exhalation through the nose. At the same time, bring your hands, palms down, in a straight line past the face, throat, heart, solar plexus, and navel, back to the starting position. Slowly flex your knees (fig. 11.4).

4. Empty your lungs with a final abdominal contraction. Pause to relax the abdominal wall. Then turn your palms upward and begin another breath (fig. 11.5).

5. You may take a short, shallow breath between the end exhalation and the beginning of the next repetition, if you wish.

175

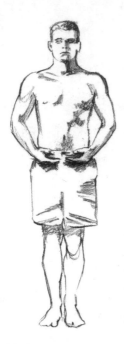

Figure 11.1

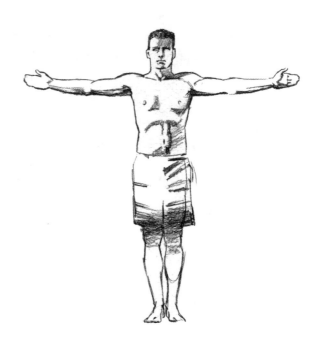

Figure 11.2

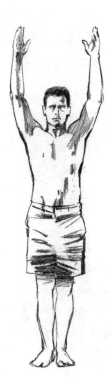

Figure 11.3

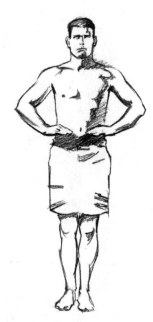

Figure 11.4

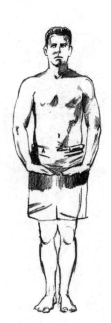

Figure 11.5

Repeat the exercise for as long as you wish, but do at least five repetitions.

 # MIND ENERGY

MEDITATION

The TriEnergetics program works because it integrates all of the body's energies. Remember, whatever affects your mind also affects your body, and vice versa.

The first week, we not only start you walking and stretching, but we start you on another vitally important part of your journey to better health. You begin a simple meditation practice.

The stress of modern life is so great and so insidious that you need to understand it in order to bring it under your control. There is an art to facing difficulties in a way that leads to effective solutions and to inner peace. It is possible to use the pressure of a problem to propel yourself through it, just as a sailor uses the pressure of the wind to move the boat through the water.

A daily practice of meditation will help you work through problems.

Ten Wonderful Benefits of Regular Meditation

> reduced heart rate

> relaxed blood vessels

> lowered blood pressure

> reduced breathing rate

> reduced oxygen intake

> decreased sweating

> reduced anxiety

> improved relaxation

> improved digestion

> enhanced immune function

Within a few weeks of beginning to meditate, you will notice changes in the way you react to unpleasant situations, and you will feel better. Trust us on this point.

How do you meditate? To review our meditation technique, refer to the Healing Light meditation exercise in chapter 8. Allow at least ten minutes every day to practice this meditation.

It is not complicated. Meditation is not about mysticism or hocus-pocus. It is about mindfulness. When you meditate, you start paying attention a little more closely to the way your mind works. You learn to be present in the moment and not fantasize about the past or the future.

What if you can't do it? At some point, you might think it foolish or boring to just sit and watch your breath going in and out. If this happens, note to yourself that this is just a thought, a judgment your mind is creating. Then let go of that thought and bring your attention back to your breathing.

If you have other thoughts, just observe them and go back to your breathing. The process of relaxation continues as long as you are sitting and breathing quietly.

If you find it too difficult to sit for ten minutes without an outside stimulus or a guide, we recommend that you get our meditation recording, available at our Web site (www.trienergetics.com). The recording will lead you through a guided relaxation.

NOURISHMENT ENERGY

SUPPLEMENTS

From the very start, we want you to use nutritional supplementation. To review our guidelines for what vitamin and mineral supplements are essential to your health, refer to the "Supplementing Sensibly" section of chapter 6.

If you are currently taking a multivitamin, it might not be adequate. Compare its ingredients against our list. You may want to make a change to a more complete formula.

EATING

The first change you need to make in your eating habits is very simple but very important. Change the foods that you snack on. Cut out all high-calorie, high-fat, nutritionally barren snack foods. You know what they are.

Snack Foods to Avoid	
› cookies	› chocolates
› cakes	› doughnuts
› muffins	› pastries
› bagels	› candy
› potato chips	› high-calorie energy bars

We have rarely met anyone who doesn't like to snack, and you are probably no exception. So by all means snack, but snack on foods that have nutritional value and are lower in calories. To make it easier to choose healthy snacks, keep a supply of sliced carrots and celery in your lunch bag and in your refrigerator. If you crave carbohydrates, try whole-grain toast rather than a doughnut or white-flour bagel.

Avoid wolfing down a high-protein energy bar before or after a workout. These bars are marketed as healthy and full of energy. In fact, "full of energy" means full of calories. Unless you work out for more than two hours a day, it is unlikely you need the additional calories or protein. More than likely, the extra calories will just be turned to fat in your body.

These foods will give you vitamins, minerals, antioxidants, and fiber, and they are also excellent snack foods. Enjoy them.

```
┌─────────────────────────────────────────────────────┐
│                  Good Snack Choices                   │
│                                                       │
│   ›  fresh fruit              ›  dried berries         │
│                                                       │
│   ›  dried fruit, such as raisins  ›  nuts             │
│      or dried cranberries                              │
│                               ›  sunflower seeds       │
│   ›  carrots                                           │
│                               ›  pumpkin seeds         │
│   ›  celery                                            │
│                               ›  whole-grain bread or toast │
│   ›  melon                                             │
│                               ›  soybeans or tofu      │
│   ›  fresh berries                                     │
└─────────────────────────────────────────────────────┘
```

Eliminating the starchy and fatty snacks will have an immediate effect on your attitude.

- You will feel better about yourself because you have taken a positive action by beginning to eat better.

- Your energy level will be better and more sustained because you will not be creating sugar highs and hypoglycemic lows.

- You will lose weight.

It may not seem like much to make such a small change in your diet, but it can pay huge dividends. Let us explain why.

The average American is about twenty pounds overweight. Since each pound is equal to about 3,500 calories, twenty pounds is the equivalent of about 70,000 calories. If you were to spread those 70,000 calories out over the course of a year, you'd find that it is only 191 calories per day of extra eating that leads to this twenty pounds of extra fat.

In other words, if you can trim only 191 calories from your diet each day, you can easily lose twenty pounds in a year. Something as small as changing your snacking habits can give you that edge to lose the weight. That's getting maximum benefit from a very simple action.

WEEKLY ACTION PLAN

You need to set goals for yourself. If you do not have a clear vision of what you want to achieve and the steps that you need to take, it won't happen; you will make a halfhearted effort and then quit in frustration. Don't let that happen.

Use the Weekly Action Plan worksheet to clarify your goals. If possible, share your action plan with your spouse or a friend. If you're working through the program by yourself, make a copy of your completed worksheet and put it in a conspicuous place to keep yourself motivated.

Weekly Action Plan: Week One

List the goals you want to achieve during the next six weeks.

_____

_____

_____

List the changes you will have to make to meet these goals.

_____

_____

_____

List the goals you would like to achieve during the next twelve months.

_____

_____

_____

List the changes you will need to make in order to reach these goals.

_____

_____

_____

That's it for week one. Remember, have fun with this. The program isn't supposed to be a punishment or a burden. It should be the beginning of a fun, active, healthy lifestyle.

Enjoy.

Week One

 ## BODY ENERGY

- Begin walking one mile at your recorded pretest time four times a week.
- Practice the Great Tai-Chi Circle Breath daily.

 ## MIND ENERGY

- Practice the Healing Light meditation for at least ten minutes every day.

 ## NOURISHMENT ENERGY

- Begin taking the recommended nutritional supplements daily.
- Eliminate high-fat, high-sugar snacks from your diet. Snack on fruits and vegetables, dried fruits, nuts, or whole-wheat toast.

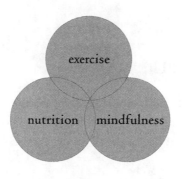

exercise

nutrition   mindfulness

chapter 12

Week Two

> For success—try aspiration, inspiration, and perspiration.
> —Satchel Paige

You've had a week to ease yourself into the program, and hopefully you are noticing some progress. The second week will move you a little farther along the path.

 BODY ENERGY

WALKING

Continue walking four times a week, paying attention to your breathing and to the sensations in your body. This week we want you to just walk a little faster. Reduce your time for the mile walk by ten seconds. As you increase your walking speed, you will improve your cardiovascular conditioning.

STRENGTH BUILDING

This week we introduce strength-building exercises into your routine. We've carefully chosen these exercises to work the major muscle groups of your abdomen, legs, chest, shoulders, and back. Working these major muscle groups

- strengthens the body

- increases endurance

- builds bone density

- improves your appearance

- increases muscle tone, which increases your metabolism so you burn more calories

- lessens low-back pain

- improves posture

Each exercise has different levels of difficulty and is illustrated and described in detail. Always begin with the easiest form of the exercise. Follow the instructions on how to do the movement and how many repetitions (reps) to do.

It is important that you exercise regularly. Do the exercises three times a week. You can choose to do them on days that you walk or on days that you don't walk. It doesn't matter.

What do you do? This week we want you to do the abdominal exercises. The purpose is to strengthen your belly muscles and your back. Strong belly muscles will improve your posture and help you get rid of that pot belly.

EXERCISE: The Isometric Crunch

The beginning form is the Isometric Crunch. It's very easy to do.

1. Lie on your back as illustrated in figure 12.1. Place your hands behind your head and bend your knees.

2. Tighten your belly muscles, but don't try to raise your shoulders off of the ground.

3. Hold the tightening for a slow count of two, then relax.

4. Do this eight times.

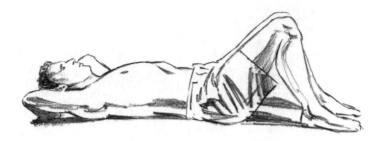

Figure 12.1

As your strength improves, add repetitions. After you can do fifteen repetitions, add a second set. Begin the second set with eight repetitions and gradually increase it to fifteen. Then add a third set. After you can do three sets of fifteen reps, you can progress to the next more difficult form, the Abdominal Crunch.

EXERCISE: The Abdominal Crunch

The Abdominal Crunch starts with the same position, but now you tense your belly muscles and lift your shoulders and upper back thirty degrees off of the ground (fig. 12.2). Hold it for one second, then relax and return to the starting position.

Once again, begin with only one set of eight reps. Progress gradually until you have worked up to three sets of fifteen reps.

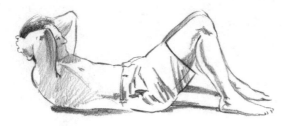

Figure 12.2

Once you can comfortably do the Abdominal Crunch, it is time to progress to the most difficult form, the One-Quarter Sit-Up.

EXERCISE: The One-Quarter Sit-Up

1. Lie on your back.

2. Elevate your legs so that both the hip and knee form a right angle (fig. 12.3).

3. Position your hands over the top of your head.

4. Raise and lower your torso quickly (fig. 12.4).

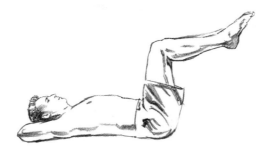

Figure 12.3

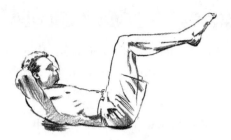

Figure 12.4

Think *up* with the torso, rather than *to the knees.* This varies the stress on the abdominals and assures greater definition of the midsection.

Once again, begin with only one set of eight reps. Progress gradually until you have worked up to three sets of fifteen reps.

How fast should you progress? Everyone will progress at a different rate. There is no need to push yourself. Remember, this is not a competition. If in the first six weeks you never progress beyond a few sets of the Isometric Crunch, you will still be making progress and will feel better.

STRETCHING

This week, add the Tai-Chi Shoulder Roll to your stretching routine. We suggest that you do the circle breath first, then move smoothly into this new stretch.

EXERCISE: The Tai-Chi Shoulder Roll

The Tai-Chi Shoulder Roll is a good way to loosen the shoulder muscles. This is the region of greatest tension for most people today.

Posture

Place your feet shoulder-width apart. Slightly bend your knees. Let your arms hang loosely down, palms facing backward. Keep your shoulders completely relaxed and slightly rounded.

Technique

1. Start rolling the shoulders up, back, down, and around (fig. 12.5).

2. Roll shoulders in as wide an arc as possible.

3. After completing ten repetitions, reverse the direction of action, rolling the shoulders forward (fig. 12.6).

4. Do another ten repetitions.

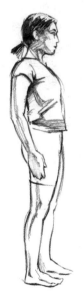
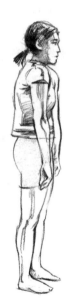

Figure 12.5   Figure 12.6

MIND ENERGY

This week, in addition to meditating ten minutes a day, we want you to wake up five minutes earlier than usual and do slow, deep abdominal breathing. Turn to chapter 9 and review the instructions for the Lying Belly Breath. Do this calming exercise for five minutes. This is a wonderful, relaxing way to start the day.

 NOURISHMENT ENERGY

This week you will make another small change in your eating habits in addition to choosing healthier snacks. We now want you to refrain from eating fatty meats.

The reason for making this change is to gradually reduce the amount of saturated animal fat in your diet. As well as promoting heart disease and weight gain, a diet high in saturated animal fat (butter, meat, and cheese) has been conclusively linked to a higher risk of cancer, including prostate cancer, ovarian cancer, and endometrial cancer.

Unacceptable High-Fat Meats and Poultry	
› bacon	› duck with skin
› marbled steak	› bologna
› lamb loin, untrimmed	› hot dogs
› beef chuck roasts, untrimmed	› braunschweiger
› beef short ribs, untrimmed	› salami
› chicken wings with skin	› smoked luncheon meats
› chicken thighs with skin	› pork sausage
	› pork spare ribs

Acceptable Low-Fat Meats and Poultry

‣ beef sirloin	‣ pork rib roast
‣ beef eye of round (select)	‣ pork chop (select)
‣ beef top round (select)	‣ pork tenderloin
‣ beef bottom round (select)	‣ extra-lean ground turkey
‣ extra-lean ground beef	‣ turkey wing
‣ trimmed porterhouse	‣ turkey breast
‣ chicken wing, no skin	‣ veal leg, top round
‣ chicken breast, no skin	‣ veal shoulder
‣ chicken thigh, no skin	‣ veal loin
‣ chicken drumstick, no skin	

When choosing meats, always choose the leanest cut. There is a huge difference in fat content between lean ground beef (80 percent fat free) and extra-lean ground beef (96 percent fat free), with no discernible difference in taste.

One serving of meat is considered to be four ounces (roughly the size of the palm of the average woman's hand). When you eat meat, limit yourself to one serving.

No more than 30 percent of your daily calories should come from fat. Eliminating these fatty meats will have a profound effect on the way you feel and will take you a long way toward getting that extra fat out of your diet.

WEEKLY ACTION PLAN

Think about the important health actions that you need to take and have been putting off. Think about the reasons that you haven't made these changes, think about the pleasures you have had by indulging in the activities that you want to change, and think about what is stopping you from taking action. Put all of your thoughts into words, and put the words onto paper. You can make a change in an instant once you are clear about what you want to do.

Weekly Action Plan: Week Two

List the important health actions that you need to take and have been putting off.

_____

_____

Why haven't you made these changes? List all of the pleasures you have received in the past by indulging in those activities that you now want to change.

_____

_____

What is stopping you from making a change? List every mental or physical obstacle to taking this positive action for yourself.

_____

_____

What is the ultimate result of not changing? Write down what it will cost you in health, image, and self-esteem if you don't take action now.

_____

_____

What are the benefits of changing? List all the pleasures you will receive by taking action now.

_____

_____

Now's the time to incorporate week two's changes into your life. Remember, no individual change is that great, but the combination of all these little changes will have a tremendous impact on your life.

Week Two

In addition to last week's practices, add the following.

 ## BODY ENERGY

- Continue to walk four times a week. This week, reduce your time by ten seconds.
- Start the abdominal exercises.
- Add the Tai-Chi Shoulder Roll to your daily stretching routine.

 ## MIND ENERGY

- Continue to do the Healing Light meditation for ten minutes each day.
- Wake up five minutes earlier each day and perform the Lying Belly Breath exercise.

 ## NOURISHMENT ENERGY

- Refrain from eating fatty meats.

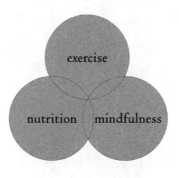

chapter 13

Week Three

> A man too busy to take care of his health is like a mechanic too busy to take care of his tools.
>
> —Spanish proverb

You have now had two weeks to work the program. Is a glimmer of excitement appearing?

Trust in the process and enjoy yourself. This is a great adventure.

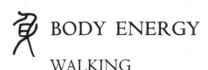 BODY ENERGY

WALKING

Continue walking four times a week, but this week, walk just a little faster. Reduce your time for the mile by another ten seconds. You will most likely find that you can lower the time by even more, but it isn't necessary. Ten seconds will do.

STRENGTH BUILDING

This week, in addition to the belly exercises, you will add leg exercises to your strength-building routine.

Your legs have the biggest and strongest muscle groups in your body and can be the source of extraordinary power. Unfortunately, in our sedentary society, the legs are often neglected. Working on your thighs will pay enormous dividends.

- stronger walking stride

- less fatigue

- better-looking butt

- increased metabolism

- stronger low back

- reduced pain and cramping in the legs

Begin with the easiest exercise, the Wall Slide, then progress to the more difficult exercises at your own pace.

EXERCISE: Wall Slide

1. Stand with your back to the wall. Place a soccer-style ball between you and the wall (fig. 13.1). The ball stabilizes your back and allows you to concentrate on the quadriceps muscles of your thighs.

2. Place your feet far enough away from the wall so that your knees will be at a ninety-degree angle when you lower your body.

3. Slowly lower your body to a count of four, then return by pushing up through the heels and midsection of the feet (not the toes) to a count of two. Breathe in as you go down and out as you go up (fig. 13.2).

Start with one set of eight repetitions. Gradually work up to fifteen reps. When that is comfortable, add a second set of eight reps. Work up to fifteen reps. Then add a third set of eight reps, working up to fifteen.

After your strength has increased, you can progress to the Full Squat.

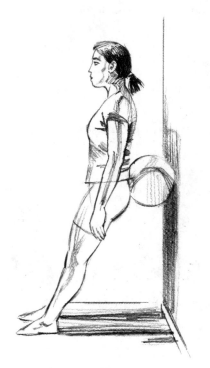

Figure 13.1

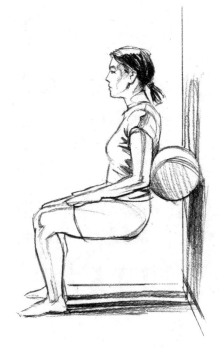

Figure 13.2

EXERCISE: Full Squat

1. Stand with your feet shoulder-width apart. Extend your arms in front of you at chest height.

2. Lower your body slowly to a count of four until your knees are at a ninety-degree angle.

3. Straighten your legs to standing to a count of two.

Begin with eight reps. Gradually work up to fifteen reps. Then add a second and third set.

When you can comfortably do three sets of fifteen reps, you can progress to the Lunges.

EXERCISE: Lunges

1. With body erect and feet shoulder-width apart (fig. 13.3), step forward (fig. 13.4) until your front knee is directly above the ankle (fig. 13.5).

2. Return by pushing off the front foot and transferring your weight back to the starting position.

3. Now step forward with the other leg.

Do eight reps, working up to fifteen reps. Then add a second and third set.

› Keep your front knee at a ninety-degree angle on the down position.

› Think more of dropping down than lunging forward.

› Dumbbells (hand weights) can be used to add more resistance.

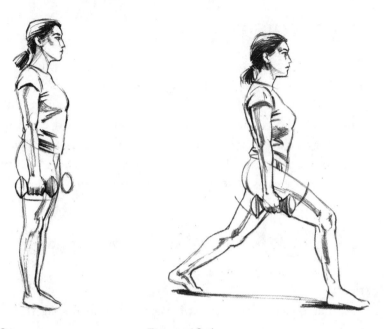

Figure 13.3

Figure 13.4

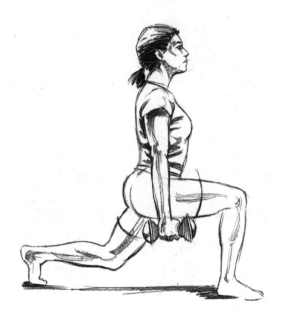

Figure 13.5

STRETCHING

This week we add the Cobra Yoga Stretch to your morning stretching routine. This move stretches and strengthens your spine and neck. Many people are plagued by stiffness in the neck, shoulders, and back. If you're one of them, you'll find this an excellent stretch to work out that stiffness.

We suggest that you add the Cobra Yoga Stretch to your routine after you've finished the Great Tai-Chi Circle Breath and the Tai-Chi Shoulder Roll. It's very nice to move smoothly from one stretch right into the next.

EXERCISE: Cobra Yoga Stretch

Posture

Lie flat on your stomach with your forehead on the floor and palms placed flat at about shoulder level, as though you were going to do a push-up (fig. 13.6).

Technique

1. Raise your head off of the ground and stretch it back until you are looking upward.

2. Then raise the top of your torso off the floor (fig. 13.7).

3. Hold this position for ten seconds, then relax.

Repeat this movement at least five times.

› Do not raise your lower abdomen off the floor, and do not straighten or lock your elbows. Don't allow your shoulders to hunch up. This is an incorrect posture (fig. 13.8).

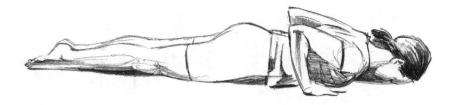

Figure 13.6

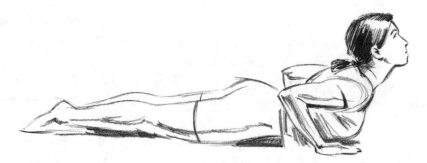

Figure 13.7

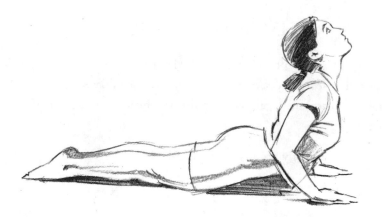

Figure 13.8

This stretch can be a bit difficult at first, so don't push it. If you feel discomfort in your back or neck, slowly let go of the stretch and rest. When you work this area gently each time you stretch, you'll find that as your back releases its tension, any discomfort will quickly fade away.

MIND ENERGY

Now that you're meditating daily and doing deep abdominal breathing every morning, we want you to apply the benefits of abdominal breathing to a common stressful situation. Many people are confronted with the everyday problems of stress while driving in traffic. It's nearly unavoidable. But you can control how your body reacts to that stressful situation.

When driving, if you feel anxious, tense, or stressed, concentrate your attention on your breath and practice deep abdominal breathing. Don't close your eyes. Just take a deep breath in, deep in the belly. Then exhale slowly. Repeat this ten times. It's easy to continue driving while calmly focusing your breath in your belly. You will be amazed at how effectively breathing relieves your anxiety and reduces your tension.

NOURISHMENT ENERGY

This week we want you to start eating at least six servings of complex carbohydrates and at least five servings of fruit and vegetables a day. Complex carbohydrates, fruits, and vegetables should be a major component of your diet. They are

- a source of vitamins and minerals

- a source of sustained energy

- relatively low in calories

- a good source of fiber

- nature's best source of antioxidants and phytochemicals

- a potent way to reduce your risk of heart disease, diabetes, and cancers

Do not pay attention to any fad diet that tells you to reduce the amount of fruit or vegetables you eat. This is simply bad advice.

You don't have to memorize serving sizes, but we've included a guide to help you gauge how much you're eating. Remember, we want you to eat at least six servings of complex carbohydrates and five servings of fruit or vegetables every day.

Serving Sizes for Fruits and Vegetables

One serving is

- one-half to one cup of raw fruit or vegetables

- one-half cup fruit or vegetable juice

- one piece of fruit

Serving Sizes for Grains, Breads, Pastas, and Starchy Vegetables

One serving is

- one slice of bread

- one-half cup hot cereal

- one cup cooked rice or pasta

- one-half to one cup cold cereal, depending on type

- one-quarter to one-half cup starchy vegetables

You can eat any fruits and vegetables you choose. For a list of the best carbohydrates choices for your daily meals—and a list of carbohydrate foods to eat only in moderation—see the "What Are Good Carbohydrate Foods?" section of chapter 4. That section also includes important guidelines about shopping for bread and cereal products.

WEEKLY ACTION PLAN

This week, think about the sources of happiness, excitement, and satisfaction in your life. Then reflect on what you are unhappy with and what changes you can make. The weekly action plan will help you to organize your thoughts.

Weekly Action Plan: Week Three

What are you happy about in your life right now?

_____

_____

What are you excited about in your life right now?

_____

_____

What are you proud of in your life right now?

_____

_____

What are you grateful for in your life right now?

_____

_____

What are you not happy about in your life right now?

_____

_____

What are you not proud of in your life right now?

_____

_____

Why are you holding on to things that are causing you unhappiness? Why are you holding on to things that you want to change? If you don't have a plan for feeling good mentally and physically, you will continue to hold attitudes and practice habits that don't work for you.

Why not make a change?

Week Three

In addition to last week's practices, add the following.

 ## BODY ENERGY

- Reduce your time for the mile by ten seconds.
- Add leg exercises to your strength routine.
- Add the Cobra Yoga Stretch to your daily stretching routine.

 ## MIND ENERGY

- Continue your practice of daily meditation.
- Practice abdominal breathing while driving.

 ## NOURISHMENT ENERGY

- Eat six servings of complex carbohydrates a day.
- Eat five servings of fruit and vegetables a day.

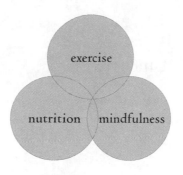

chapter 14

Week Four

> You are never too old to become younger.
>
> —Mae West

You are now halfway through the program. Look back and see how far you have come. Remember, it all began with one small step.

 BODY ENERGY

WALKING

This week, increase your walking speed and reduce your one-mile time by another ten seconds.

STRENGTH BUILDING

In addition to the abdominal and leg exercises, you will begin an exercise designed to work the muscles of your chest, your arms, and your shoulders.

EXERCISE: Chest Press

The Chest Press requires the use of elastic exercise bands. You can purchase these bands at most sporting goods stores or through our Web site at www.trienergetics.com.

1. Begin with the easiest band.

2. Put the band behind your back and grab the handles in front of you (fig. 14.1).

3. Slowly straighten your arms to a count of four (fig. 14.2).

4. Then relax to a count of two.

Breathe in as you relax and out as you straighten your arms.

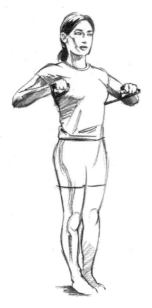

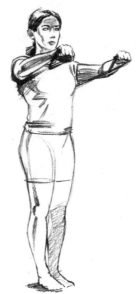

Figure 14.1   Figure 14.2

Begin with eight repetitions. Gradually increase to fifteen repetitions. Then add a second and third set.

STRETCHING

Now we add the Tai-Chi Chest Expander Stretch to your daily routine. This move works very well in concert with the Chest Press exercise; together they will help stretch and strengthen the chest.

EXERCISE: Tai-Chi Chest Expander

This stretch works to loosen the shoulders and back, preparing the body for deep breathing.

Posture

Stand comfortably with your knees slightly bent and your arms in front of you with palms down (fig. 14.3).

Technique

1. Swing your arms out to the sides, turning your palms upward, until your arms reach the full limit of the stretch (fig. 14.4). Keep your arms parallel to the ground throughout the stretch.

2. Then swing them back in front, turning your palms downward.

Breathe in as your arms swing open, out as you return.
Do at least twenty repetitions.

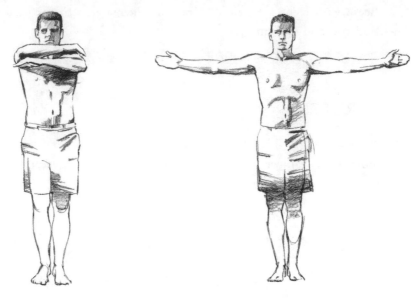

Figure 14.3   Figure 14.4

 MIND ENERGY

In addition to meditating daily and practicing abdominal breathing in the morning and when you're driving, we want you to experiment with mindful eating.

Remember that mindful eating helps you recognize when you have had enough to eat, when your appetite has been satisfied, and when you are no longer hungry. Mindful eating is also very calming. It is a unique form of meditation.

Pick a quiet time when you are alone and won't be disturbed. While practicing mindful eating, do not read, talk, or watch television. Concentrate on each and every bite of food you place in your mouth. Slow down your eating. Pay attention to the flavor and the texture. Chew slowly and purposefully. Notice the sensations in your body when you chew and when you swallow. Breathe deeply between bites.

For more detailed instructions about mindful eating, see chapter 5.

NOURISHMENT ENERGY

This week, in addition to the eating changes you made during the first three weeks, we want you to become less of a meat eater.

Even lean meat is high in saturated fats and cholesterol and contains hormones, antibiotics, and pesticides. Many studies conclusively link high meat consumption with high rates of cancer of the breast, prostate, uterus, pancreas, kidney, rectum, and colon.

Two-thirds of your daily protein should come from plant sources. In addition to being lower in fat and calories, these foods are significant sources of antioxidants, vitamins, and fiber not found in meats.

It isn't necessary to become a vegetarian unless you want to. If you crave a steak or a slice of roast beef, you don't have to give it up. We only ask that you eat less red meat. Limit yourself to lean red meat and eat it no more than three times a week.

WEEKLY ACTION PLAN

This week, think about everything you would like to do to improve your mental and physical health. List these things in order of priority, and set a timeline for achieving each goal. Remember, if you don't set goals for yourself, you will get stuck where you are.

Choose your most important goal from the list. Write a short statement about why you are absolutely committed to achieving this goal.

Weekly Action Plan: Week Four

Write down everything that you would like to improve that relates to your personal, mental, and physical health.

_____

_____

Give yourself a timeline for achieving each goal.

_____

_____

Choose your most important goal from the list.

_____

Write a paragraph or two about why you are absolutely committed to achieving this goal.

_____

_____

_____

_____

_____

_____

_____

_____

_____

_____

_____

Nothing can stop you from reaching your goal except yourself. Why not take control over your life now? Remember, some people succeed because they are destined to, but most of us succeed because we are determined to.

Week Four

In addition to last week's practices, add the following.

 ## BODY ENERGY

- Lower your time for the mile by ten seconds.
- Add the Chest Press to your strength routine.
- Add the Tai-Chi Chest Expander to your stretching routine.

 ## MIND ENERGY

- Continue to meditate daily.
- Practice mindful eating.

 ## NOURISHMENT ENERGY

- Refrain from fatty meats, and eat lean red meat no more than three times a week.

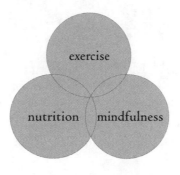

chapter 15

Week Five

> There is more to life than increasing its speed.
>
> —Mahatma Gandhi

You have passed the halfway mark and are heading down the home stretch. You should be noticing that your body is getting stronger and that your endurance is increasing. Feels good, doesn't it?

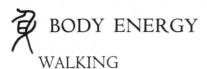 BODY ENERGY

WALKING

Continue walking a mile four times a week. This week, try to lower your time for the mile by another ten seconds.

STRENGTH BUILDING

Many people develop a chronic low backache as they get older. This week you will add a low-back exercise to your routine. This exercise will strengthen your lower back and also improve your posture. Begin with the Prone Extension.

EXERCISE: The Prone Extension

1. Lie facedown with your feet slightly apart, back relaxed, and arms extended in front of you (fig. 15.1).

2. Keeping your head down, hips and abdominals tightened, lift one of your legs and your opposite arm (fig. 15.2).

3. Hold for five seconds. Repeat five times on each side to make one set.

When you can comfortably complete one set, add a second and then a third set. When you can comfortably complete three sets, it is time to move on to the next exercise.

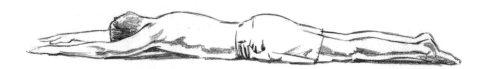

Figure 15.1

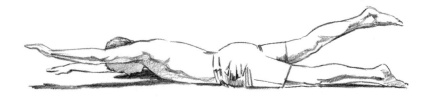

Figure 15.2

EXERCISE: The Quadriped

1. Get on your hands and knees, keeping knees directly under hips and hands directly under shoulders (fig. 15.3).

2. Keeping your hips level and abdominals tight, extend one leg until it is parallel to the floor (fig. 15.4). Hold for five seconds, then switch sides.

3. Repeat the exercise five times per side to make one set.

Once you can do this easily, add a second and third set. Once you can perform three sets, move to the Advanced Quadriped, where you extend one leg and the opposite arm simultaneously (fig. 15.5).

› Keep abdominals tight at all times while performing this exercise.

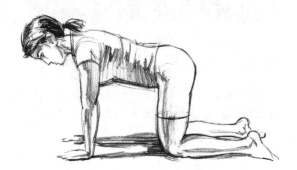

Figure 15.3

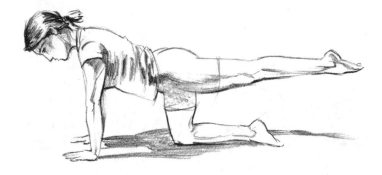

Figure 15.4

217

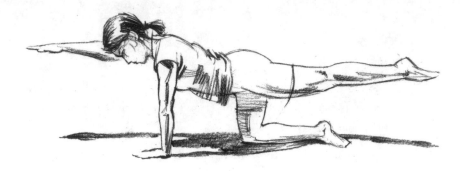

Figure 15.5

EXERCISE: The Bridge

It would be a good idea to have someone watch you the first few times you do this exercise to be certain you are doing it properly.

1. Lie on your back on the floor with back flat, palms on the floor, knees bent, and feet flat on the floor (fig. 15.6).

2. Place a pillow under your head.

3. Contract your abdominal and buttock muscles. Lift your hips until there is a straight line from your knees to your shoulders (fig. 15.7). Hold for five seconds, then relax.

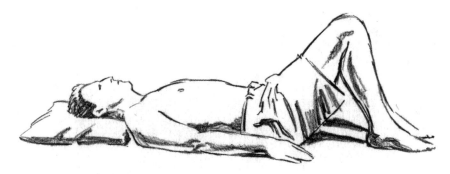

Figure 15.6

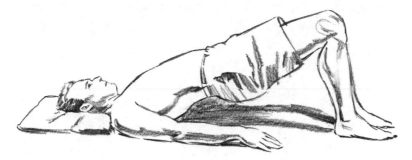

Figure 15.7

Repeat the sequence. When you can complete ten reps, add a second set, working up to ten reps. Then add a third set.

STRETCHING

The new stretch this week is the Tai-Chi Spine and Torso Twist. This beautifully complements the new low-back exercise to limber and strengthen your lower back.

EXERCISE: Tai-Chi Spine and Torso Twist

Posture

Stand comfortably with your knees slightly bent and your shoulders and arms as relaxed as possible.

Technique

1. Using only your thighs, twist your torso slowly left, then right (fig. 15.8 and 15.9).

2. Gently increase the twist, allowing your arms to swing out from the centrifugal force.

219

3.   As soon as the twist in one direction is complete, start turning the other way.

Do 15 reps.

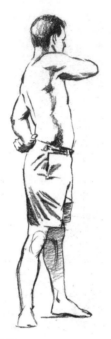
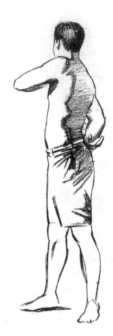

Figure 15.8   Figure 15.9

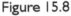

 MIND ENERGY

This week you will again focus on one of the major stresses in modern life: driving. Most people push their time to the limit. Consequently, they are always running late and frantically trying to catch up. They speed through traffic, run yellow lights, and curse at other drivers, all because they are running behind.

In addition to meditating daily and practicing abdominal breathing, we want you to make a commitment to reducing your daily level of driving-related stress. This may sound hard, but you can do it easily.

Our suggestion is simple. When you have to drive someplace (to an appointment, to a meeting, to pick up a child), we want you to leave for your destination fifteen minutes earlier. That's it. The extra time you have will dramatically reduce your travel-related stress.

NOURISHMENT ENERGY

This week, in addition to the eating changes you have made during the first four weeks, we're going to move you a little farther away from your reliance on eating meats. We want you to eat two vegetarian dinners per week.

You may already be eating some meals without any red meat, chicken, or fish. But if you always have some kind of meat or fish with your meals, this will be an important change.

Vegetarian meals can be very appealing and very tasty. You have unlimited choices. A good whole-grain pasta meal, like spinach pasta with eggplant and a red wine tomato sauce, counts as a vegetarian dinner.

You will learn that to feel satisfied, you don't have to eat meat at every meal.

WEEKLY ACTION PLAN

This week we want you to think about your hindrances. These are the traits that keep you from getting where you want to go. The weekly action plan will help give you some insight into how to get past these blocks and move forward to achieve your goals.

Weekly Action Plan: Week Five

Make a list of the hindrances that are keeping you from successfully achieving your goals.

_____

_____

_____

_____

_____

_____

Look over your list. Isn't it possible to progress past these blocks? What do you need to do?

_____

_____

_____

_____

_____

_____

_____

Week Five

In addition to last week's practices, add the following.

 BODY ENERGY

- Reduce your time for the mile by ten seconds.
- Add low-back exercises to your strength routine.
- Add the Tai-Chi Spine and Torso Twist to your stretching routine.

 MIND ENERGY

- Continue to meditate daily.
- Leave for your destination fifteen minutes early to reduce traffic-related stress.

 NOURISHMENT ENERGY

- Eat at least two vegetarian dinners per week.

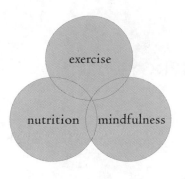

exercise

nutrition | mindfulness

chapter 16

Week Six

May you live all the days of your life.

—Jonathan Swift

You started the TriEnergetics program with a single small step, but after five weeks, you have taken giant strides on the path toward better health and a new you.

If you have followed all parts of the program, you will have noticed remarkable changes in your energy level and in the way that you feel. You may also have noticed that you are handling stressful situations much better than before. Hasn't it been remarkably easy?

These five weeks are only a beginning. Take the lessons you have learned and continue working the program. There is no limit to what you can achieve.

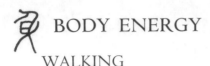

BODY ENERGY

WALKING

This week, reduce your walking time for a mile by another ten seconds.

STRENGTH BUILDING

This week you will add an upper back exercise to the abdominal, lower-back, chest, and leg exercises.

EXERCISE: Latissimus Strengthener

This exercise will help develop your latissimus muscles and the other muscles of your upper back. Begin with the easiest elastic band and progress at your own rate.

1. Grasp the handles of the elastic band with palms facing each other. Extend your arms above your head (fig. 16.1).

2. Gradually pull your hands away from each other, keeping your arms straight at the elbow (fig. 16.2).

3. Continue pulling your arms down until they are parallel with the floor (fig. 16.3).

4. Relax and slowly allow the arms to return to the overhead position.

5. Pull down to a count of four and return to a count of two.

6. Breathe out as you go down, in as you go up.

Start with eight repetitions, working up to fifteen repetitions. Then add a second set and a third. When you can comfortably do three sets of fifteen reps, move to the harder band. Begin the progression with one set of eight reps, working up to three sets of fifteen reps.

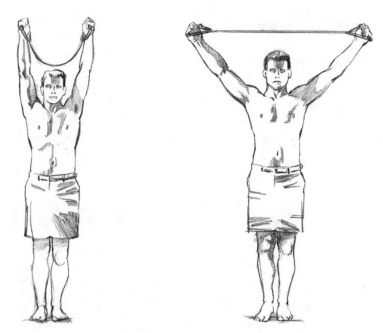

Figure 16.1   Figure 16.2

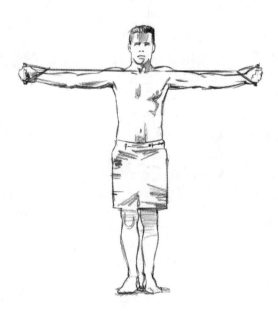

Figure 16.3

STRETCHING

This week you'll add the Tai-Chi Upper-Back Loosener to your stretching routine.

You, like many people, may store chronic stress and fatigue in the muscles of your upper back. This exercise helps to combat stiffness and nicely complements the Latissimus Strengthener exercise to strengthen and loosen the muscles of the upper back.

EXERCISE: Tai-Chi Upper-Back Loosener

Posture

- Stand erect with your heels together and toes pointed out at forty-five degrees.

- Relax your arms, reach back, and clasp your hands behind your back with your palms together, interlacing your fingers.

Technique

1. Stretch your neck up, roll your shoulders backward, and try to bring your elbows as close together as possible (fig. 16.4).

2. Hold the position for a count of six, then relax and repeat three times.

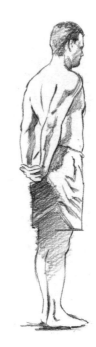

Figure 16.4

MIND ENERGY

We want you to expand your use of abdominal breathing. It is an incredibly powerful tool to help you relax and get centered.

In addition to meditating daily and practicing abdominal breathing for five minutes in the morning and when stressed in traffic, we suggest that several times a day, you relax for a minute or two. Close your eyes, breathe into your belly, and allow the tension to leave your muscles. You can do this while at your desk at work, at home, or on a break. These short breaks will refresh you and reenergize you.

 NOURISHMENT ENERGY

This week we want you to take the next step toward lowering the fat and cholesterol in your diet.

From now on, eat only fat-free dairy products, and limit yourself to no more than two eggs a week. If you really like omelets, try egg-white omelets or omelets made with one complete egg and only the whites of one or two others.

WEEKLY ACTION PLAN

This week, think deeply about the changes you have observed in yourself since you started the program.

Weekly Action Plan: Week Six

List the changes that you have observed in yourself.

_____

_____

_____

_____

List the changes that you wanted to make but that haven't happened yet.

_____

_____

_____

_____

Why haven't they happened? Can you list any reasons you have not been successful in making these changes?

_____

_____

_____

_____

List ways you can get motivated to make these changes happen.

_____

_____

_____

_____

Week Six

In addition to last week's practices, add the following.

BODY ENERGY

- Reduce your time for the mile by ten seconds.
- Add the Latissimus Strengthener to your strength routine.
- Add the Tai-Chi Upper-Back Loosener to your stretching routine.

MIND ENERGY

- Continue to meditate daily.
- Practice deep abdominal breathing several times a day while at home or work.

NOURISHMENT ENERGY

- Eat only fat-free dairy products.
- Eat no more than two eggs a week.

Congratulations!

You have completed the first six weeks of the TriEnergetics program. You are on your way to a healthier you. Continue your good work and enjoy your success.

We've included a posttesting sheet for you to fill out. This will give you an idea of some of the progress you've made during the six weeks. Remember, most of your progress—how you feel, how you handle stress, and your sense of well-being—cannot be adequately measured on a form. Look inside yourself to see how you may have changed in these areas.

The path to wellness isn't a quick or simple one. It is a lifetime commitment. We trust that you have learned many valuable techniques, exercises, and facts that you can use on your continued journey. We hope you've been encouraged enough by your success these last six weeks to continue on the path.

We will be there for you as you carry on with your journey, even after you've completed the first six weeks. Contact us whenever you feel the need or if you have questions, through our Web site at www.trienergetics.com.

With peace and well-being, we wish you continued success.

TriEnergetics Program Posttesting

Date: _____

Resting heart rate _____ Blood pressure _____

Blood cholesterol _____ Weight _____

Measurements: Arms _____ Chest _____ Waist _____

            Hips _____ Thighs _____

Timed one-mile walk _____ Heart rate after one-mile walk _____

Comments: _____

_____

_____

_____

_____

_____

_____

_____

chapter 17

The Path Awaits

We invite you to do something for yourself. Experiment with the program. Make a positive change for yourself.

Experiment with living intentionally from moment to moment. By that, we mean try to live in the present moment and don't dwell on the failures you had—or think you have had—in the past. For the purpose of what you are doing now, the past does not matter.

You will succeed. Set your goals and put your judgmental mind to rest. Changes will occur in a very natural way, and we know you will be delighted by your progress.

Trust the process of change and try to let go of your resistance to giving up habits that you know are not healthy. We know this is difficult.

CATCHING MONKEYS

Eastern philosophers address the mind's difficulty letting go of its set ways by using the metaphor of catching monkeys.

As the story goes, in ancient days, hunters used coconuts to catch monkeys. They'd cut a hole in the coconut just big enough for a monkey to put its hand through. Then they'd secure the coconut to the base of a tree, put a banana inside the coconut, and hide. With time, the monkey would come down, put its hand in the coconut, and grab the banana.

Now here's the trick. The hole would be just small enough so that the open hand could go in, but the clenched hand with the banana could not get out. To get free, all the monkey needed to do was to let go of the banana. But most monkeys wouldn't let go.

WE'RE NOT MONKEYS

In spite of all of our intelligence, in many ways humans behave just like those monkeys. Our minds just don't want to let go of our old self-destructive habits and ways. We get caught in a trap of our own making.

TriEnergetics will help you get free. Not only that, but with time and patience, you'll arrive at a new awakening.

The program will work if you work the program.

Be well.

References

Bingham S. A., N. E. Day, R. Luben, P. Ferrari, N. Slimani, T. Norat, F. Clavel-Chapelon, E. Kesse, A. Nieters, H. Boeing, A. Tjonneland, K. Overvad, C. Martinez, M. Dorronsoro, C. A. Gonzalez, T. J. Key, A. Trichopoulou, A. Naska, P. Vineis, R. Tumino, V. Krogh, H. B. Bueno-de-Mesquita, P. H. Peeters, G. Berglund, G. Hallmans, E. Lund, G. Skeie, R. Kaaks, and E. Riboli. 2003. Dietary fibre in food and protection against colorectal cancer in the European Prospective Investigation into Cancer and Nutrition (EPIC): An observational study. *Lancet* 361 (9368): 1496–501.

Chao, A., M. J. Thun, and C. J. Connell. 2005. Meat consumption and risk of colorectal cancer. *Journal of the American Medical Association* 293 (2): 172–82.

Fitness fact: Burn more calories. 1998. *Senior Times,* March.

Friedman, E. H. 1994. Morning and Monday: Critical periods for the onset of AMI. *European Heart Journal* 15 (12): 1727.

Goel, M. S., E. P. McCarthy, R. S. Phillips, and C. C. Wee. Obesity among U.S. immigrant subgroups by duration of residence. *Journal of the American Medical Association* 292 (23): 2860–7.

Jin, P. 1989. Changes in heart rate, noradrenaline, cortisol, and mood during tai chi. *Journal of Psychosomatic Research* 33 (2): 197–206.

Kagan, A. 1996. *The Honolulu Heart Program: An Epidemiological Study of Coronary Heart Disease and Stroke.* Amsterdam: Harwood Academic.

Liu, S., J. E. Buring, H. D. Sesso, E. B. Rimm, W. C. Willet, and J. E. Manson. A prospective study of dietary fiber intake and risk of cardiovascular disease among women. *Journal of the American College of Cardiology* 39 (1): 49–56.

Manson, J. E., P. H. Greenland, A. Z. LaCroix, and M. L. Stefanick. 2002. Walking compared with vigorous exercise for the prevention of cardiovascular events in women. *New England Journal of Medicine* 347 (10): 716–25.

Olsen, A. K., E. M. Bladbjerg, A. K. Hansen, and P. Marckmann. A high-fat meal activates blood coagulation factor VII in rats. *Journal of Nutrition* 132 (3): 347–50.

Olshansky, S. J., D. J. Passaro, R. C. Hershow, J. Layden, B. A. Carnes, L. Hayflick, R. N. Butler, D. B. Allison, and D. S. Ludwig. A potential decline in life expectancy in the United States in the twenty-first century. *New England Journal of Medicine* 352 (11): 1138–45.

Paffenbarger, R. S., Jr., and I. M. Lee. 1997. Intensity of physical activity related to incidence of hypertension and all-cause mortality: An epidemiological view. *Blood Pressure Monitoring* 2 (3): 115–123.

Peters, U., R. Sinha, N. Chatterjee, A. F. Subar, R. G. Ziegler, M. Kulldorff, R. Bresalier, J. L. Weissfeld, A. Flood, A. Schatzkin, and R. B. Hayes. 2003. Dietary fibre and colorectal adenoma in a colorectal cancer early detection programme. *Lancet* 361 (9368): 1487–8.

Rosenman, R. H., R. J. Brand, C. D. Jenkins, M. Freidman, R. Straus, and M. Wurm. 1975. Coronary heart disease in the Western Collaborative Group Study: Final follow-up experience of eight and a half years. *Journal of the American Medical Association* 233:872–7.

Samaras, K., P. J. Kelly, M. N. Chiano, T. D. Spector, and L. V. Campbell. 1999. Genetic and environmental influences on total-body and central abdominal fat: The effect of physical activity in female twins. *Annals of Internal Medicine* 130 (11): 873–82.

Smith, E. L., Jr., P. E. Smith, C. L. Ensign, and M. M. Shea. Bone involution decrease in exercising middle-age women. *Calcified Tissue International* 36 suppl 1:S129–38.

Tsang, C., S. Higgins, G. G. Duthie, S. J. Duthie, and M. Howie. 2005. The influence of moderate red wine consumption on antioxidant status and indices of oxidative stress associated with CHD in healthy volunteers. *British Journal of Nutrition* 93 (2): 233–40.

Weinsier, R. L. 1999. Genes and obesity: Is there reason to change our behaviors? *Annals of Internal Medicine* 130 (11): 938–9.

Woodward, T. S., H. Tunstall-Pedoe, and C. Bolton-Smith. 1999. Fiber and heart disease. *American Journal of Epidemiology* 150 (10): 1073–80.

Wu, H. 2005. A case study of type 2 diabetes self-management. *Biomedical Engineering Online* 4:4 (doi 10.1186/1475-925x-4-4).

Sanford L. Severin, MD, is an internationally renowned physician and assistant professor at the University of California, San Francisco. He has lectured extensively throughout the world, having delivered several hundred invited lecture presentations. His lectures have been televised in Europe, and he has been featured twice on Dr. Dean Edell's syndicated medical television show. While serving in the Air Force at the Aerospace Medical Center in the 1960s, he worked extensively with the nation's first Apollo astronauts as part of a team evaluating their mental and physical fitness. He began a twenty-year study of meditation in the 1970s and has continued this pursuit of Vapassana training with noted author and teacher, Steven Levine. Severin is a fitness enthusiast, former collegiate wrestler, and life-long student of Eastern philosophy.

Todd D. Severin, MD, began his study of the mind/body relationship at Pomona College. He received national recognition for creating his major field of study, behavioral biology, the integration of the human mind and body. He studied tai chi and Taoist healing with world-renowned Taoist master, Abraham Liu. Severin serves as lecturer at Meiji College of Oriental Medicine in San Francisco, and is assistant clinical professor at the University of California, Berkeley, School of Optometry. He is the author of medical articles, and chapters in books, and has received awards for his scientific research. He is a highly sought after speaker, having presented over two hundred lectures across the United States, Europe, and Asia. His seminars have been televised throughout California, and he has been a featured guest on the cable health show Community Health and the radio feature Health Issues.